AF147571

Dermatology High-Yield Self-Assessment

Sima Jain

Dermatology High-Yield Self-Assessment

Supplement to Dermatology: Illustrated Study Guide and Comprehensive Board Review

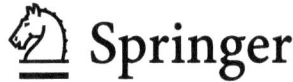 Springer

Sima Jain
Department of Dermatology
University of Florida College of Medicine
Gainesville, Florida, USA

ClearSkin Dermatology
Private Practice
Orlando, Florida, USA

ISBN 978-3-031-73262-1   ISBN 978-3-031-73263-8   (eBook)
https://doi.org/10.1007/978-3-031-73263-8

© The Editor(s) (if applicable) and The Author(s), under exclusive license to Springer Nature Switzerland AG 2024
This work is subject to copyright. All rights are solely and exclusively licensed by the Publisher, whether the whole or part of the material is concerned, specifically the rights of translation, reprinting, reuse of illustrations, recitation, broadcasting, reproduction on microfilms or in any other physical way, and transmission or information storage and retrieval, electronic adaptation, computer software, or by similar or dissimilar methodology now known or hereafter developed.
The use of general descriptive names, registered names, trademarks, service marks, etc. in this publication does not imply, even in the absence of a specific statement, that such names are exempt from the relevant protective laws and regulations and therefore free for general use.
The publisher, the authors and the editors are safe to assume that the advice and information in this book are believed to be true and accurate at the date of publication. Neither the publisher nor the authors or the editors give a warranty, expressed or implied, with respect to the material contained herein or for any errors or omissions that may have been made. The publisher remains neutral with regard to jurisdictional claims in published maps and institutional affiliations.

This Springer imprint is published by the registered company Springer Nature Switzerland AG
The registered company address is: Gewerbestrasse 11, 6330 Cham, Switzerland

If disposing of this product, please recycle the paper.

I would like to dedicate this book to Dr. Stanton Wesson, my first dermatology mentor, whom I met as a medical student at the University of Florida Department of Dermatology in Gainesville, Florida. Dr. Wesson was an amazing dermatologist with incredible skill, expertise, and bedside manner. He taught me the importance of always striving for excellence in both clinical acumen and bedside manner. His passing was an incredible loss to our field but his legacy carries forward with all of the medical students and dermatology residents hementored over the years. He was one of the smartest, most dedicated, and passionate dermatologists I have ever met, and I will always be grateful for the time we had together and the knowledge he bestowed upon me.

Preface

This dermatology board self-assessment book is an invaluable tool for any dermatologist wishing to test and improve their knowledge of dermatology. It includes over 350 multiple-choice questions, along with over 180 high-quality color images that cover the full breadth of the specialty using clinical vignettes that test not only the readers' knowledge but also the ability to apply that knowledge in clinical practice. It serves as a supplement to *Dermatology: Illustrated Study Guide and Comprehensive Board Review* and follows the same outline of chapters including medical, surgical, and cosmetic dermatology. The questions are intended to highlight the important teaching points that are both clinically relevant and high yield.

Orlando, FL, USA   Sima Jain MD

Acknowledgment

I would like to thank the staff at Springer, particularly Lee Klein and Michelle Tam. You both have been incredible to work with. Lee, thank you for being so meticulous and organized throughout this process. Michelle, thank you for your tireless efforts in helping me find the best clinical images for this book. I will always be grateful to both of you for all of your help.

Contents

1. **In normal hair cycling, what is the approximate percentage of hair follicles in the anagen phase?**
   (a) 50–60%
   (b) 80–95%
   (c) 70–80%
   (d) 95–100%

2. **Which of the following is the correct order of the different concentric layers of hair from innermost to outermost?**

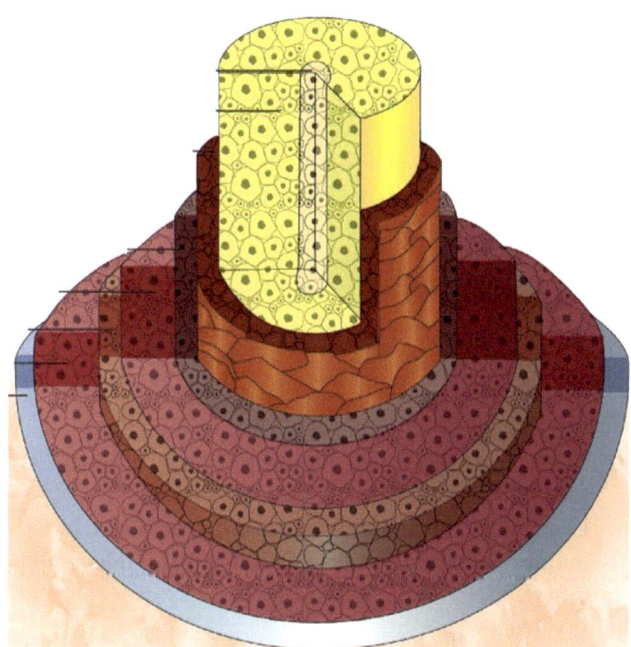

   (a) Medulla → Cortex → Cuticle (part of inner root sheath [IRS]) → Huxley (IRS) → Henle (IRS) → Outer root sheath (ORS)
   (b) Cortex → Medulla → Henle (IRS) → Huxley (IRS) → Cuticle (IRS) → ORS
   (c) Medulla → Cortex → Cuticle (IRS) → Henle (IRS) → Huxley (IRS) → ORS
   (d) Cortex → Medulla → Cuticle (IRS) → Huxley (IRS) → Henle (IRS) → ORS

3. **Scalp hair grows approximately how many centimeters per month?**
   (a) 0.2 cm
   (b) 1.2 cm
   (c) 2.5 cm
   (d) 0.5 cm

4. **An excision within the nail bed should be oriented longitudinally, while an excision within the nail matrix should be oriented horizontally.**
   (a) True
   (b) False

5. **The dorsal aspect of nail plate is created by the distal nail matrix while the proximal matrix is responsible for producing the undersurface of the nail plate, and thus to minimize permanent nail dystrophy, a biopsy should be performed in the proximal matrix when possible.**

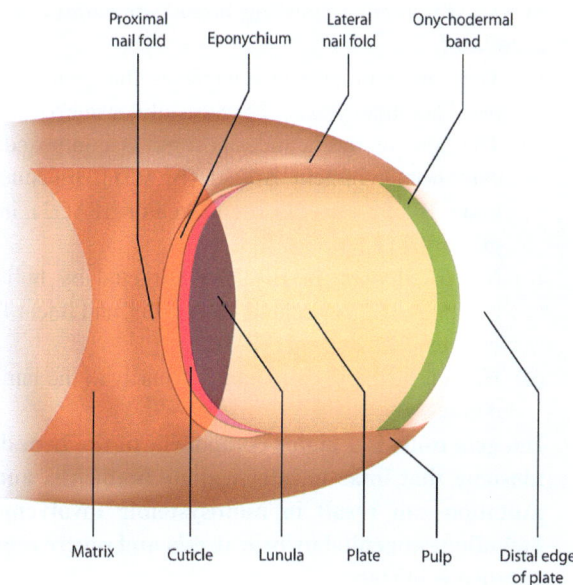

   (a) True
   (b) False

© The Author(s), under exclusive license to Springer Nature Switzerland AG 2024
S. Jain, *Dermatology High-Yield Self-Assessment*, https://doi.org/10.1007/978-3-031-73263-8_1

6. **Which of the following is NOT true regarding the nail apparatus?**

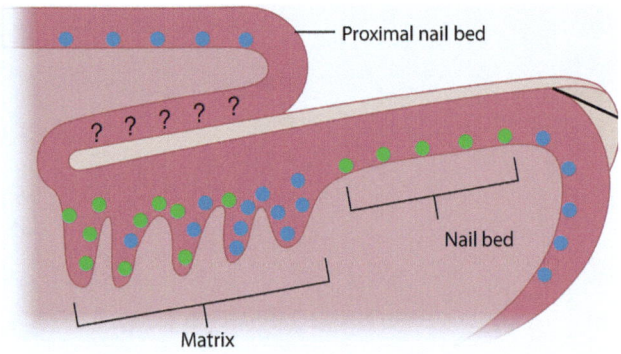

(a) Melanocytes in the proximal matrix are typically dormant and do not produce melanin pigment

(b) Melanocytic activation is the most frequent cause of benign melanonychia in adult patients

(c) The lunula demarcates the distal portion of the nail matrix

(d) Complete replacement of the fingernail requires approximately 12 months

7. **Which of the following statements is the most accurate regarding laminin-332?**

(a) It is a major cell surface receptor for epidermal adhesion to the basement membrane

(b) A mutation in laminin-332 is seen in recessive dystrophic epidermal bullosa (RDEB)

(c) A mutation causes mucous membrane pemphigoid (MMP) with an increased risk of malignancy

(d) It is a major component of anchoring fibrils

8. **Which statement regarding hemidesmosomes is not accurate?**

(a) They are multiprotein complexes that help attach basal keratinocytes to the extracellular matrix

(b) The core of the hemidesmosome is composed of cytoplasmic protein BP230 (BPAG1), transmembrane BP180 (type XVII collagen or BPAG2), integrin α6β4 and plectin

(c) NC16A domain of BP230 is targeted by bullous pemphigoid, pemphigoid gestationis, and linear IgA bullous dermatosis (LABD)

(d) Hemidesmosomes are found primarily in the lamina densa

9. **Integrin α6β4 is a major component of the hemidesmosome that links to intermediate filaments, and a mutation can result in multisystemic involvement including congenital pyloric atresia and severe mucocutaneous blisters.**

(a) True

(b) False

10. **In addition to epidermolysis bullosa, a mutation in plectin may result in muscular dystrophy because plectin can be found not only in epithelia and fibroblasts but also in muscle.**

(a) True

(b) False

11. **Which of the following statement is the most accurate regarding mutations involving the basement membrane zone components?**

(a) Integrin α6β4 is a cellular adhesion molecule that binds laminin in the extracellular matrix, and a mutation can result in junctional epidermolysis bullosa with muscular dystrophy

(b) Plectin is a cytoskeletal protein that maintains tissue integrity, and a mutation may cause junctional epidermolysis bullosa with pyloric atresia (JEB-PA)

(c) Type VII collagen is the main component of anchoring fibrils, and a mutation may cause dystrophic epidermolysis bullosa (DEB)

(d) Laminin-332 is a major component of anchoring filaments and a mutation causes epidermolysis bullosa simplex (EBS)

12. **The following are all true regarding type III collagen except which statement?**

(a) Type III collagen dominates the early phase of wound healing along with granulation tissue formation

(b) Type III collagen is typically replaced by stronger type I collagen in wound healing

(c) Type III collagen is more common in fetal skin

(d) A mutation in type III collagen results in the vascular form of Ehlers-Danlos syndrome

(e) It is the most abundant type of collagen found in the human body

13. **A defect in Type VII collagen is involved in all of the following except:**

(a) Epidermolysis bullosa acquisita (EBA)

(b) Bullous systemic lupus erythematosus (SLE)

(c) Recessive dystrophic epidermolysis bullosa (RDEB)

(d) Junctional epidermolysis bullosa (JEB)

14. **Located in the stratum corneum, urocanic acid is a major epidermal chromophore for ultraviolet radiation (UVR).**

(a) True

(b) False

15. **Which of the following statements about loricrin is the least accurate?**

(a) Loricrin is the predominant protein of the cornified cell envelope

(b) A mutation causes the classic form of Vohwinkel syndrome

(c) Loricrin is located in keratohyaline granules (KHGs) within the granular layer

(d) Loricrin found within KHGs terminally differentiate to form a cornified cell envelope

16. **Increased filaggrin expression contributes to the deficient epidermal barrier formation seen in atopic dermatitis, and a mutation in the gene has been identified as the cause of lamellar ichthyosis.**
    - (a) True
    - (b) False

17. **The average number of days for epidermal turnover is approximately:**
    - (a) 10 days
    - (b) 30 days
    - (c) 50 days
    - (d) 120 days

18. **Eccrine glands are found in the following location:**
    - (a) Glans penis
    - (b) Clitoris
    - (c) Labia minora
    - (d) Labia majora

19. **"Free" sebaceous glands (not associated with hair follicles) include the following locations except:**
    - (a) Superficial eyelid margin (Glands of Zeis)
    - (b) Nipple and areola (Montgomery tubercles)
    - (c) Tarsal plate of eyelids (Meibomian glands)
    - (d) External fold of prepuce (Tyson's glands)
    - (e) Vermilion border of lips and buccal mucosa (Fordyce spots)
    - (f) Nail bed (Brunner's glands)

20. **Which of the following is the least likely cause of mast cell activation?**
    - (a) Sudden change in temperature, heat, and/or cold
    - (b) Stress
    - (c) Alcohol
    - (d) Exercise
    - (e) Tetracyclines (i.e., doxycycline)
    - (f) Nonsteroid anti-inflammatory drugs (NSAIDs)
    - (g) Infection
    - (h) Mechanical friction of the skin

21. **All of the following are preformed mast cell mediators except:**
    - (a) Histamine
    - (b) Chymase
    - (c) Prostaglandin D2
    - (d) Tryptase
    - (e) Carboxypeptidase A

22. **Neuroendocrine markers found within Merkel cells include all of the following except:**
    - (a) Thyroid transcription factor 1 (TTF-1)
    - (b) Neuron-specific enolase (NSE)
    - (c) Chromogranin-A
    - (d) Synaptophysin
    - (e) Protein gene product (PGP) 9.5

23. **The electron micrograph shown here is a picture of what structure?**

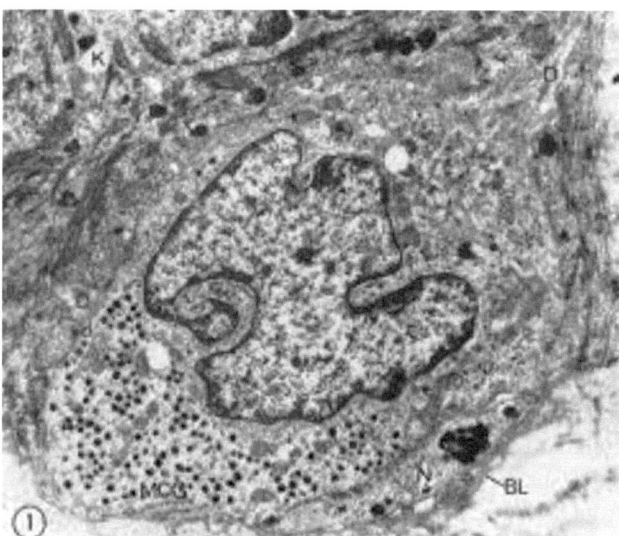

    - (a) Birbeck granule from Langerhans cell
    - (b) Electron-dense granules seen in Merkel cells
    - (c) Electron-dense granules seen in mast cells
    - (d) Curved tonofilaments in squamous cell carcinoma
    - (e) Clumped tonofilaments in epidermolysis bullosa simplex, variant Dowling-Meara

24. **The following arrow in the electron microscopy picture shows what structure?**

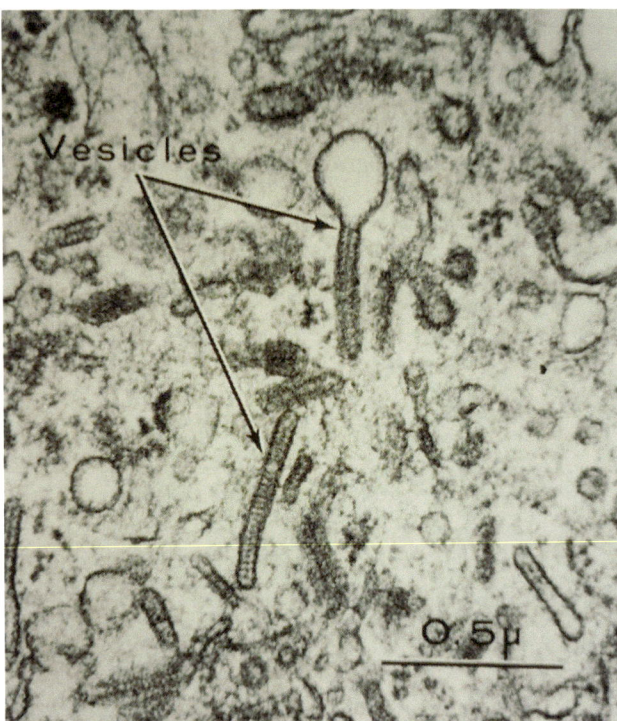

   (a) Clumped tonofilaments
   (b) Birbeck granules
   (c) Mast cell granules
   (d) Hemidesmosomes

25. **Which of the following is not an accurate statement regarding melanin and melanocytes?**
   (a) Eumelanin and pheomelanin are the two types of melanin in skin, hair, and eyes
   (b) Pheomelanin is the dark brown pigment, while eumelanin is a yellow to red pigment and associated with increased susceptibility to free radical damage from UV irradiation
   (c) The ratio of melanocytes to keratinocytes is approximately 1:10 in the epidermal basal layer
   (d) The epidermal-melanin unit composed of one melanocyte and approximately 36 neighboring keratinocytes in the epidermal basal layer

26. **Binding of melanocortin-stimulating hormone (MSH) to melanocortin 1 receptor (MC1R) switches pigment from pheomelanin to eumelanin, and MC1R mutations (such as CDKN2A and CDK4) have been shown to increase the risk of cutaneous melanoma.**
   (a) True
   (b) False

27. **The number of melanocytes in human skin of all types is essentially the same, but darker skinned patients have melanosomes that are larger, oval-shaped, and denser, while light skinned patients have smaller and less dense melanosomes clustered in membrane-bound groups.**
   (a) True
   (b) False

28. **Toll-like receptors (TLRs) are an important part of adaptive immunity, and each TLR recognizes a different pathogen-associated molecular pattern (PAMP) on microorganisms.**
   (a) True
   (b) False

29. **Topical imiquimod is a synthetic analogue of:**
   (a) Toll-like receptor 2
   (b) Toll-like receptor 3
   (c) Toll-like receptor 4
   (d) Toll-like receptor 5
   (e) Toll-like receptor 7

30. **The C1 inhibitor is a protease inhibitor that blocks the complement system, and a deficiency of this results in the unchecked production of vasodilator bradykinin (resulting in angioedema).**
   (a) True
   (b) False

31. **Which of the following is not an accurate statement?**
   (a) Type 2 immunity is considered central to atopic dermatitis pathogenesis and key therapeutic agents
   (b) IL-4 and IL-13 are both pivotal cytokines involved in the generation of allergic disease
   (c) The role of Th1 cell differentiation and Th1 cytokines is central to the pathogenesis of psoriasis
   (d) Proinflammatory Th1 cytokines include IFN-γ, IL-12, IL-23, and IL-17
   (e) Dupilumab is an IgG4 human monoclonal antibody (mAb) that binds IL-13

32. **Interleukin (IL)-17 is a proinflammatory cytokine that links T cell activation to neutrophil mobilization and activation.**
   (a) True
   (b) False

33. **Which of the following is the least accurate regarding phosphodiesterase-4 (PDE4)?**
    (a) It is an intracellular enzyme that degrades cyclic adenosine monophosphate (cAMP)
    (b) Inhibition of phosphodiesterase-4 results in increased intracellular cAMP levels
    (c) Increased cAMP levels result in decreased inflammatory mediators such as TNF-α, IFN- γ, IL-12, and IL-23
    (d) Increased cAMP levels also increase the production of anti-inflammatory mediators such as IL-2
    (e) Apremilast inhibits PDE-4

34. **HLA (human leukocyte antigen) B27 is associated with which of the following disease(s)?**
    (a) Ankylosing spondylitis, reactive arthritis, and psoriatic arthritis
    (b) Behçet's disease
    (c) Psoriasis
    (d) Celiac disease, dermatitis herpetiformis

35. **HLA-Cw6 is associated with which of the following disease(s)?**
    (a) Anklyosing spondylitis, reactive arthritis, psoriatic arthritis
    (b) Behçet's disease
    (c) Psoriasis
    (d) Celiac disease, dermatitis herpetiformis

36. **HLA-DQ2 is associated with which of the following disease(s)?**
    (a) Anklyosing spondylitis, reactive arthritis, and psoriatic arthritis
    (b) Behçet's disease
    (c) Psoriasis
    (d) Celiac disease and dermatitis herpetiformis

37. **HLA-B51 is associated with which of the following disease(s)?**
    (a) Anklyosing spondylitis, reactive arthritis, psoriatic arthritis
    (b) Behçet's disease
    (c) Psoriasis
    (d) Celiac disease, dermatitis herpetiformis

Answer Key

For further information regarding the below answers, please see Chapter 1 of the corresponding *Dermatology: Illustrated Study Guide and Comprehensive Board Review, third Edition* (2024).

1. **b**
2. **a**
3. **b**
4. **a**
5. **b**
6. **d**
7. **c**
8. **d**
9. **a**
10. **a**
11. **c**
12. **e**
13. **d**
14. **a**
15. **b**
16. **b**
17. **c**
18. **d**
19. **f**
20. **e**
21. **c**
22. **a**
23. **b**
24. **b**
25. **b**
26. **a**
27. **a**
28. **b**
29. **e**
30. **a**
31. **e**
32. **a**
33. **d**
34. **a**
35. **c**
36. **d**
37. **b**

Image Sources

1.2 Anastassakis, K. (2022). The Morphology and Structure of the Hair Shaft. In: Androgenetic Alopecia From A to Z. Springer, Cham. https://doi.org/10.1007/978-3-030-76111-0_6

1.5 González-Serva, A. (2018). Normal Nail Anatomy, Normal Nail Histology, and Common Reaction Patterns. In: Rubin, A.I., Jellinek, N.J., Daniel, C.R., Scher, R.K. (eds) Scher and Daniel's Nails. Springer, Cham. pp. 39–82. https://doi.org/10.1007/978-3-319-65649-6_4

1.6 Fleckman, P., McCaffrey, L. (2018). Structure and Function of the Nail Unit. In: Rubin, A.I., Jellinek, N.J., Daniel, C.R., Scher, R.K. (eds) Scher and Daniel's Nails. Springer, Cham. https://doi.org/10.1007/978-3-319-65649-6_5

1.23 Kidd, R.L., Krawczyk, W.S. & Wilgram, G.F. The Merkel cell in human epidermis: its differentiation from other dendritic cells. Arch. Derm. Forsch. 241, 374–384 (1971). https://doi.org/10.1007/BF00595269

1.24 Wikipedia. Birbeck granules. https://en.wikipedia.org/wiki/Birbeck_granules (CC BY-SA 2.0) https://creativecommons.org/licenses/by-sa/2.0/

1. This eruption was seen at birth in a full-term baby. A smear of the pustule would show which of the following?

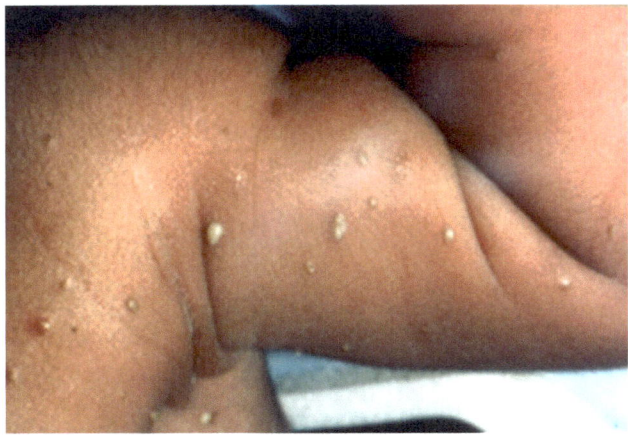

(a) Neutrophils
(b) Eosinophils
(c) No cells
(d) Needle-shaped clefts

2. Which of the following statements is the *least accurate* regarding spinal dysraphism?
(a) It is defined as incomplete fusion of midline mesenchymal, bony or neural elements of the spine
(b) Both the skin and nervous tissue are of ectodermal origin, so anomalies may occur in both simultaneously
(c) Occult spinal dysraphism (OSD) is seen when neural tissue is covered with skin, making the diagnosis less apparent
(d) A lipoma in a baby over the lumbosacral region may be a marker of occult spinal dysraphism and warrants further evaluation
(e) A solitary small dimple over the lumbosacral region is a strong indicator of occult spinal dysraphism and always warrants imaging even if it is an isolated finding

3. The following abnormality is seen in this baby. Which of the findings below would be least likely associated with an underlying closure defect of the cranial neural tube?

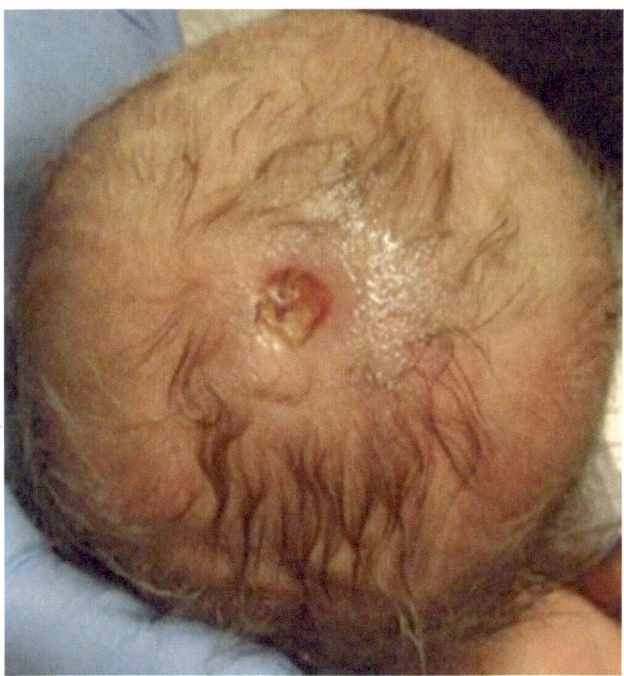

(a) Coarse or long hairs encircling aplasia cutis congenita (ACC)
(b) Large ulcerative ACC that appears fluid-filled
(c) Small hairless atrophic ACC
(d) Location at the midline of the vertex

© The Author(s), under exclusive license to Springer Nature Switzerland AG 2024
S. Jain, *Dermatology High-Yield Self-Assessment*, https://doi.org/10.1007/978-3-031-73263-8_2

4. **What is the concern when seeing a child with this lesion over the lumbosacral region at birth?**

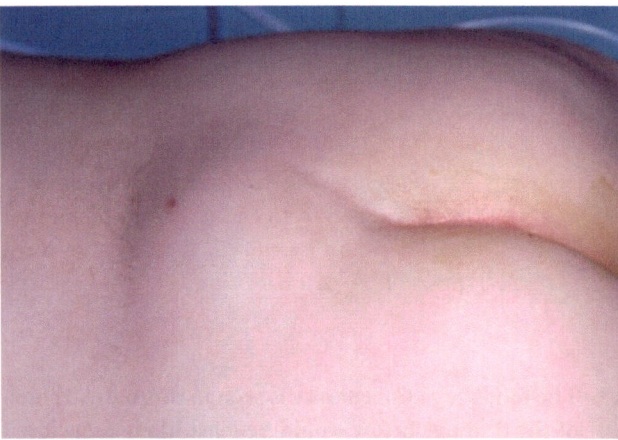

    (a) Underlying spinal dysraphism and therefore an MRI is indicated

    (b) No imaging is needed as there is no concern if it is an isolated finding

    (c) Potential malignant transformation and therefore the area should be carefully monitored

5. **What may be associated with this healthy baby at 2 weeks of age seen with indurated subcutaneous nodules to the buttocks and thighs?**

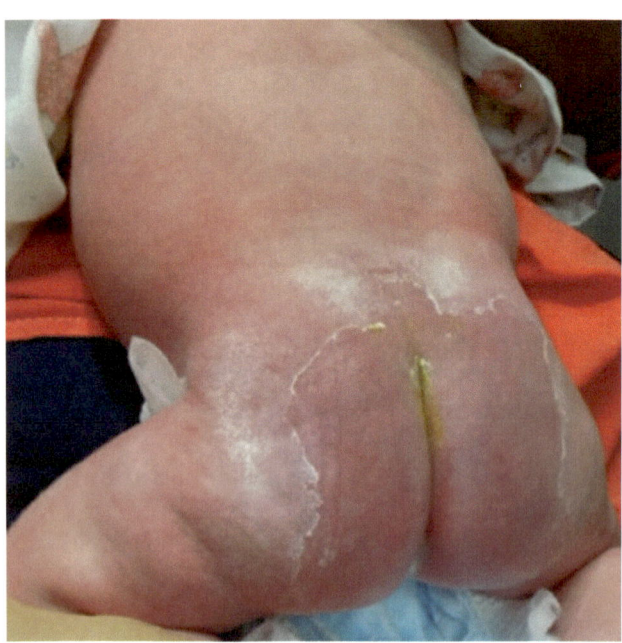

    (a) Occult spinal dysraphism

    (b) Hypercalcemia

    (c) Heart failure

    (d) Polycythemia

    (e) Thrombocythemia

6. **The following rash was preceded by vesicles along the leg of an infant. What is the most likely diagnosis?**

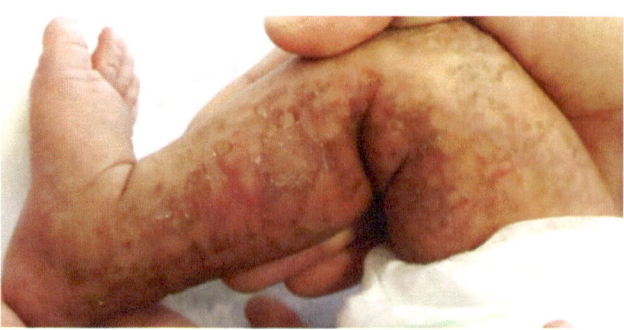

    (a) Incontinentia pigmenti

    (b) Cutis marmorata

    (c) Epidermal nevus

    (d) Lichen striatus

7. **Which of the following features would be the least likely to be seen in a baby with the following blaschkoid plaques on the extremities and lateral torso?**

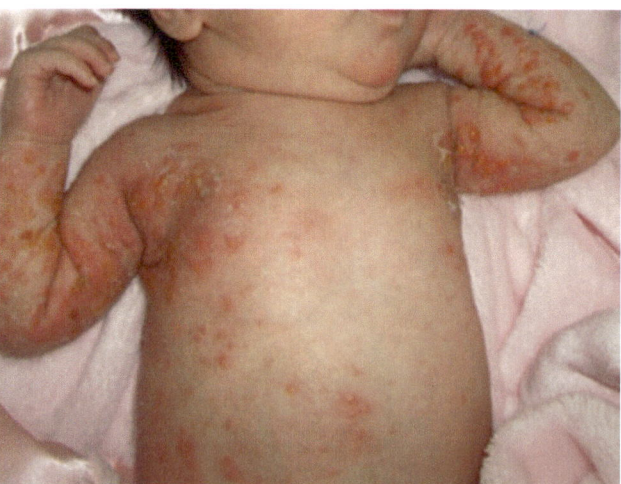

    (a) Ocular abnormalities

    (b) CNS abnormalities (i.e., seizures or delayed psychomotor development)

    (c) Patchy scarring alopecia

    (d) Absent or peg-shaped teeth

    (e) Thrombocytopenia

8. **Which of the following is the least accurate statement regarding the condition shown in the figure?**

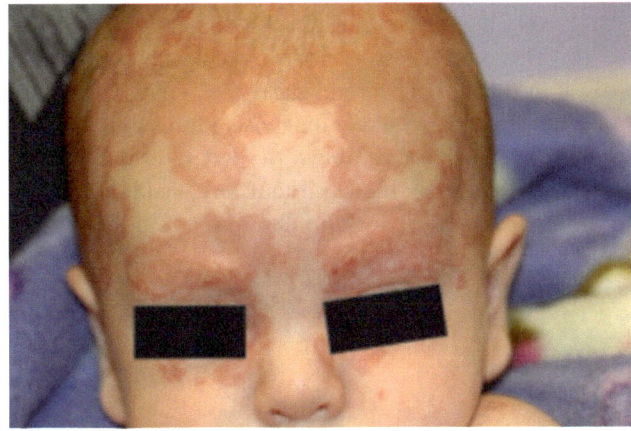

(a) It is a subtype of lupus erythematosus
(b) The most serious sequela is immune-mediated congenital heart block
(c) Approximately, 50% will have complete heart block at presentation
(d) Exposure of the developing atrial-ventricular node (AVN) in the fetus to the maternal Ro/La antibodies lead to local inflammation and potential permanent scarring of the AVN, resulting in inability to transmit the heart rhythm from the atrium to the ventricle

9. **What is the most accurate statement regarding this 6-month-old baby with a periorificial and perianal rash?**

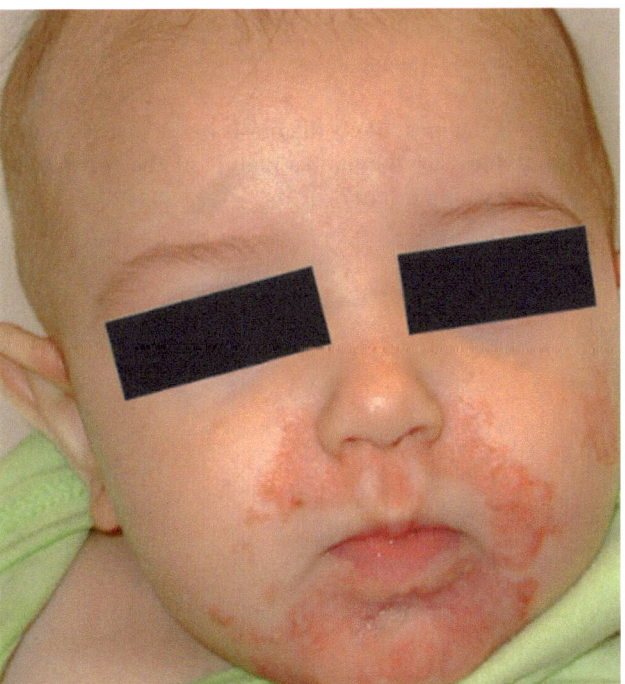

(a) It is most likely due to decreased bioavailability of zinc in manufactured milk, unlike breast milk and often seen when infants wean off breast milk
(b) It is due to excess bioavailability of zinc found in manufactured milk and seen when premature infants wean off breast milk
(c) It is related to a severe deficiency of niacin (B3)
(d) It is due to a deficiency in vitamin A and accompanied by foamy silver-gray spots on the conjunctiva called Bitot spots

10. **What is the concern in this baby with a firm mass with overlying telangiectasias that has suddenly become enlarged and painful?**

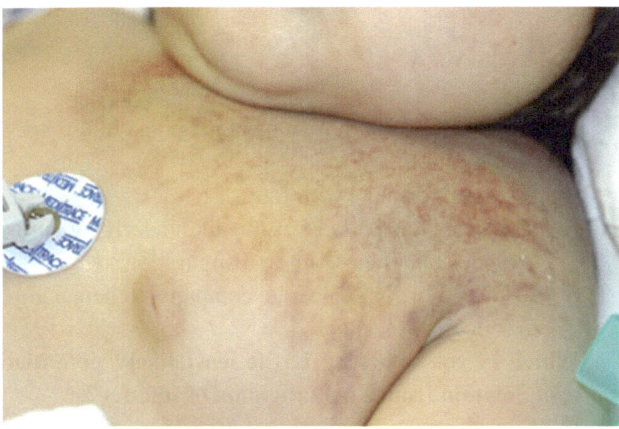

(a) Hemangiomas in internal organs causing heart failure and jaundice
(b) Entrapment and destruction of platelets resulting in thrombocytopenia and coagulopathy
(c) Ulceration and pain to the site
(d) Underlying hypocalcemia, pain, and scarring to the site

11. **What is most accurate statement regarding a hemangioma involving the nasal tip?**

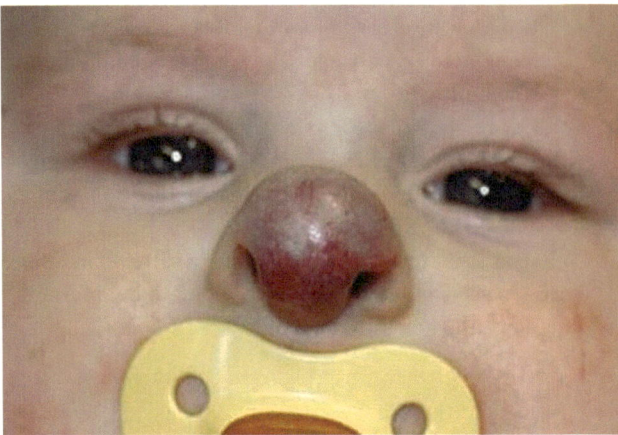

   (a) It is much harder to treat a hemangioma in this specific location
   (b) It will not involute with time
   (c) The hemangioma may distort the underlying cartilage and can often result in disfiguration
   (d) It is more likely to ulcerate compared to hemangiomas in other locations

12. **Which of the following is the least likely potential complication from a hemangioma of infancy?**
   (a) Congestive heart failure (if visceral hemangiomas, especially in liver)
   (b) Obstructive jaundice (especially if liver involved)
   (c) Laryngeal hemangiomatosis with potential airway obstruction (especially if involving the beard region)
   (d) Restrictive cardiomyopathy if involving cardiac tissue

13. **What is the most accurate statement for the following lesion?**

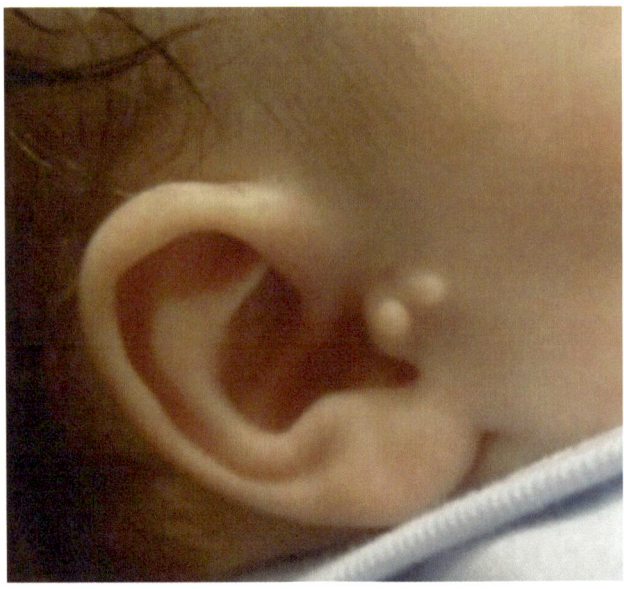

   (a) This is a branchial cleft remnant and a solitary lesion is not indicative of any genetic problem or syndrome
   (b) This marks the entrance to a sinus tract that has a very high rate of infection
   (c) This is an accessory parotid gland with extension to the underlying parotid gland

14. **What is the most likely diagnosis in this child with a slow-growing lesion above the left lateral eyebrow, found soon after birth without any visible punctum and negative for transillumination?**

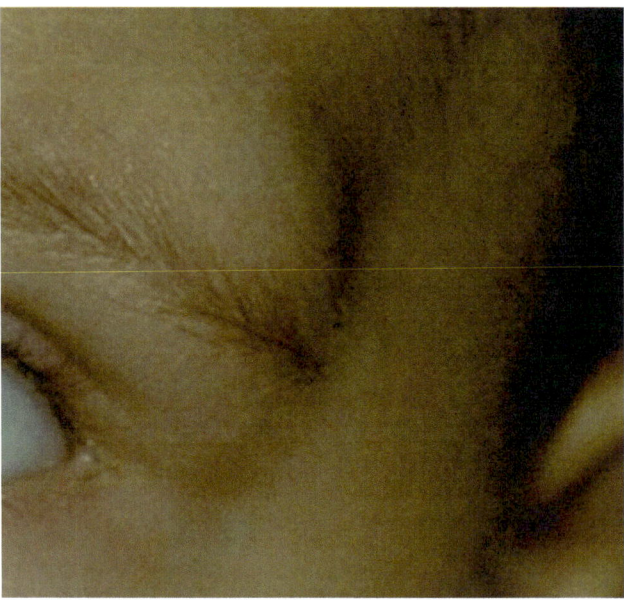

   (a) Branchial cleft cyst
   (b) Encephalocele
   (c) Thyroglossal duct cyst
   (d) Dermoid cyst

15. **What is the most likely diagnosis in the picture showing a shiny, erythematous nodule of the third right toe in a young infant?**

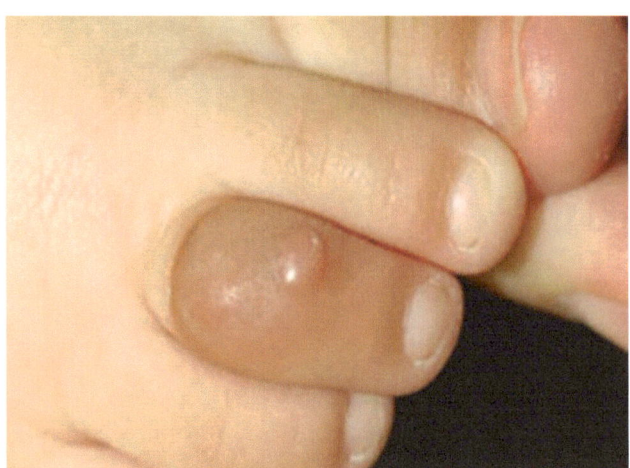

(a) Multicentric reticulohistiocytosis
(b) Infantile digital fibroma
(c) Fibrosarcoma
(d) Chondrosarcoma

16. **What is the most likely diagnosis in this baby with the following lesion on the cheek and the associated histopathology picture?**

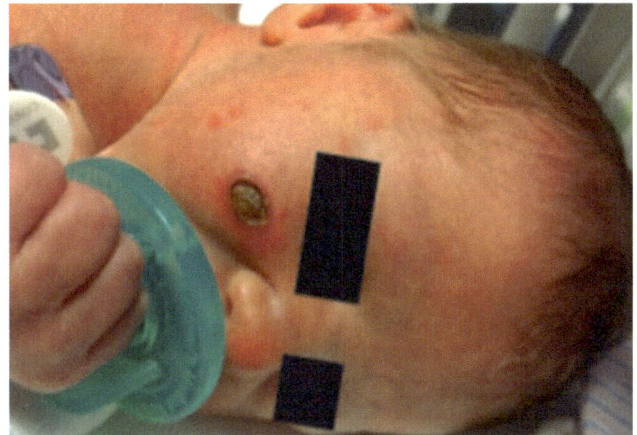

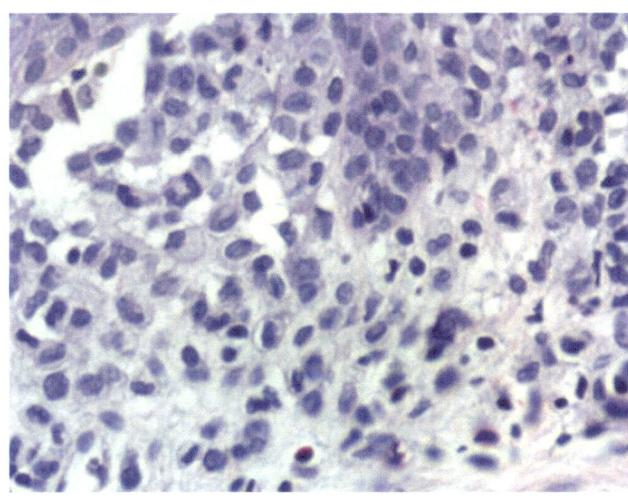

(a) Langerhans cell histiocytosis
(b) Ecthyma
(c) "Popsicle" panniculitis
(d) Discoid lupus erythematosus

17. **What is the least accurate statement regarding neurocutaneous melanosis?**
    (a) It is characterized by the presence of congenital melanocytic nevi (CMN) and benign or malignant melanocytic tumors of the central nervous system
    (b) It may result in increased intracranial pressure, seizures, developmental delay, cranial nerve palsies, hypotonia, and spinal cord compression
    (c) Imaging with an MRI is helpful to rule out neurocutaneous melanosis

(d) There is a high risk of CMN associated with neurocutaneous melanoma if large sized congenital melanocytic nevus with multiple satellite lesions
(e) There is a low risk for neurocutaneous melanosis with CMN if the location is within the posterior axis (head, neck and paravertebral regions)

18. **The most likely diagnosis in this 2-year-old child pictured with brown to red papules that form a wheal when stroked is likely which of the following?**

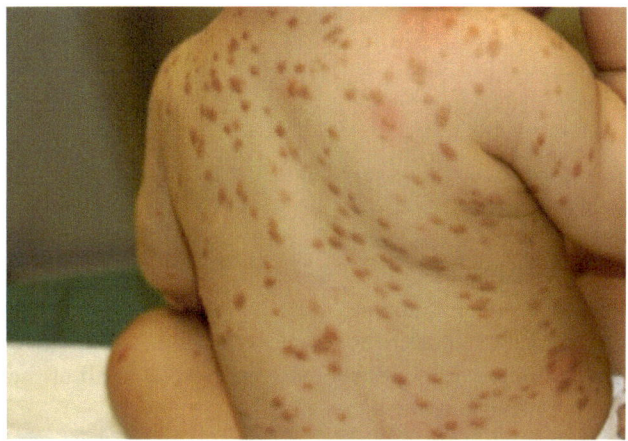

(a) Urticaria pigmentosa
(b) Benign cephalic histiocytosis
(c) Langerhans cell histiocytosis
(d) Multiple juvenile xanthogranulomas

19. **Multiple pilomatricomas can be seen in which of the following conditions?**

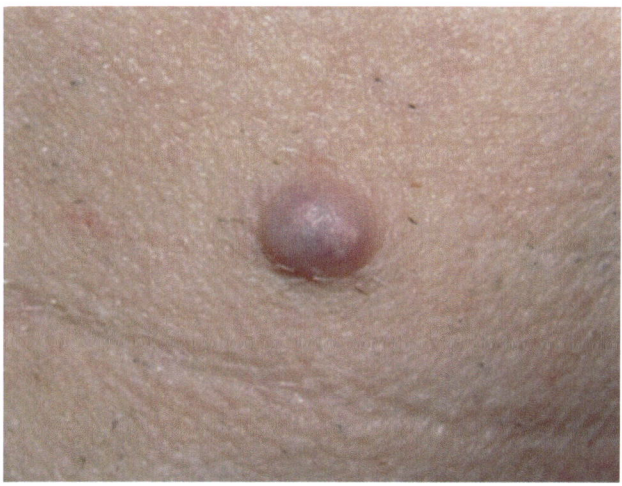

(a) Tuberous sclerosis
(b) Brooke-Spiegler syndrome
(c) Myotonic dystrophy
(d) Gardner syndrome

20. **What is the most likely diagnosis of this patient with waxy, reddish-brown papules primary distributed along the central face?**

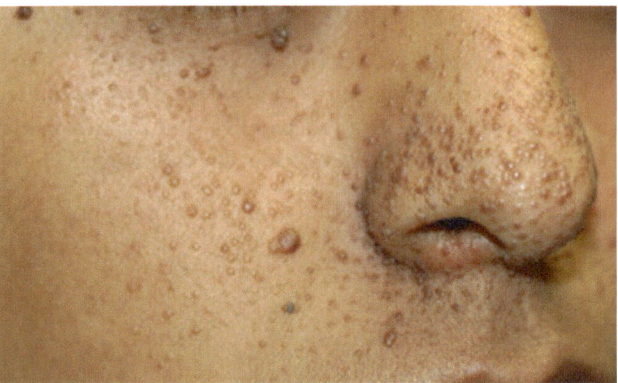

   (a) Cowden syndrome
   (b) Brooke-Spiegler syndrome
   (c) Gardner syndrome
   (d) Tuberous sclerosis complex

21. **Multiple trichoepitheliomas can be seen in all of the following except?**

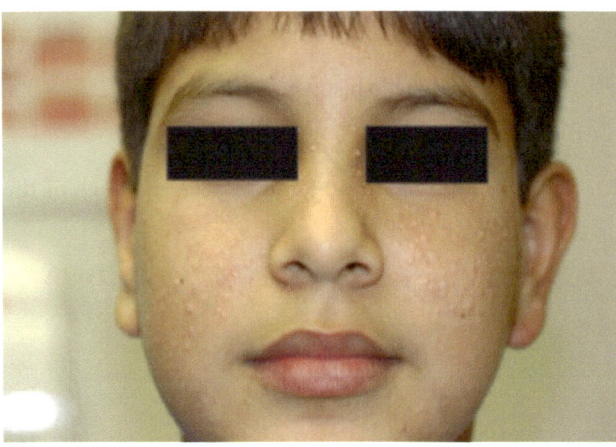

   (a) Brooke-Spiegler syndrome
   (b) Rombo syndrome
   (c) Multiple familial trichoepitheliomas
   (d) Rasmussen syndrome
   (e) Cowden syndrome

22. **The most likely diagnosis in this child with a verrucous alopecic plaque on the vertex on the scalp that used to be smooth is most likely which of the following?**

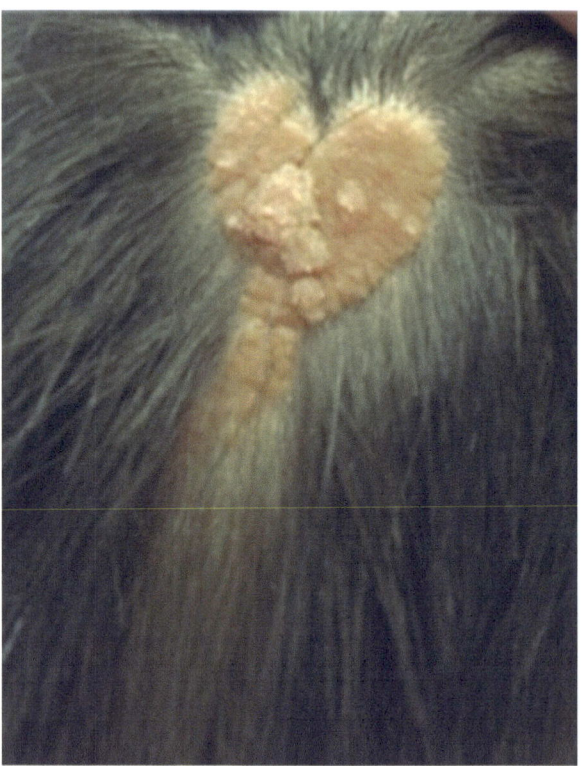

   (a) Nevus sebaceous
   (b) Epidermal nevus
   (c) Collagenoma
   (d) Aplasia cutis congenita

23. **What is the most likely diagnosis in this 4-year-old child whose parents noticed a lack of hair at the temporal hairline for the past 2 years? It has not changed in size during this time. On dermoscopic examination, you see vellus hairs throughout the area and no evidence of scarring. She has no history of similar lesions in the past.**

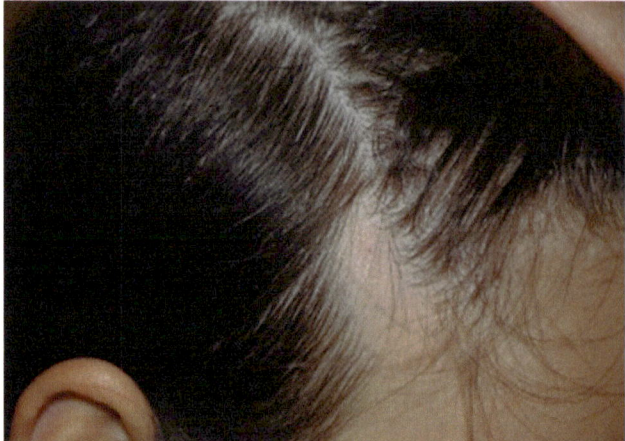

   (a) Congenital triangular alopecia
   (b) Alopecia areata
   (c) Trichotillomania
   (d) Tinea capitis

24. **What is the most likely diagnosis of this 6-month-old baby with a low-grade fever and rash pictured in the figure?**

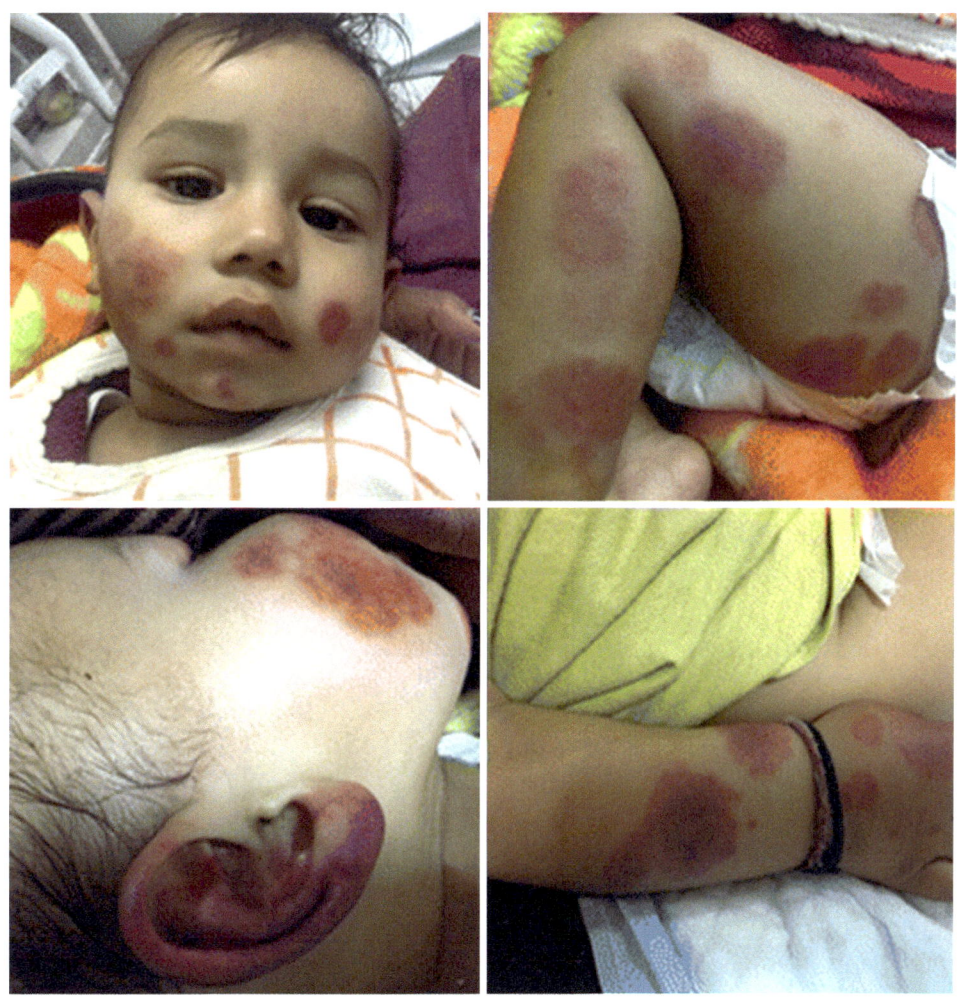

   (a) Papular purpuric gloves and socks syndrome
   (b) Erythema infectiosum or fifth disease
   (c) Atopic dermatitis
   (d) Periorificial granulomatous dermatitis
   (e) Acute hemorrhagic edema of infancy

25. **What would you be the most concerned about in a child (under the age of 5) with abdominal pain, fever, conjunctival injection, cervical lymphadenopathy, edema with desquamation of the hands and feet, and edematous lips with a red tongue?**

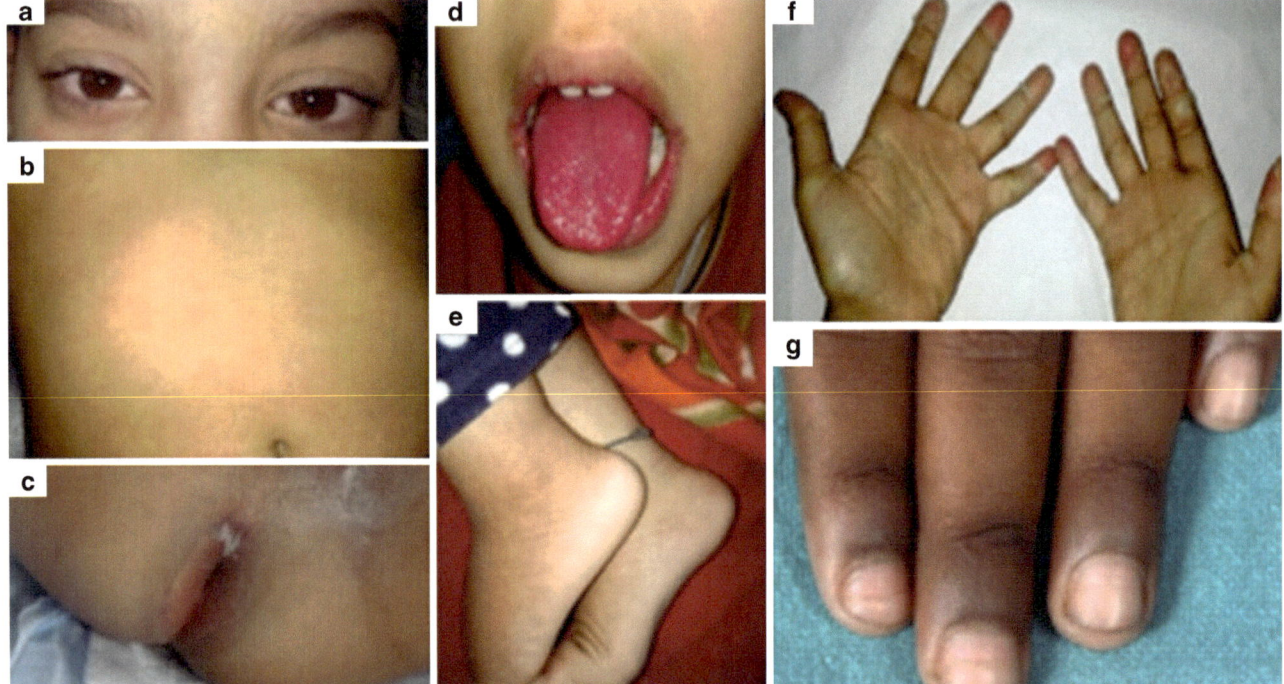

(a) Myocarditis and potential cardiac aneurysm
(b) Leukocytoclastic vasculitis
(c) Seizures
(d) Encephalitis
(e) Gastrointestinal bleed

26. **What is the most likely diagnosis in this 8-year-old girl with an asymptomatic rash on the left cheek for 6 months?**

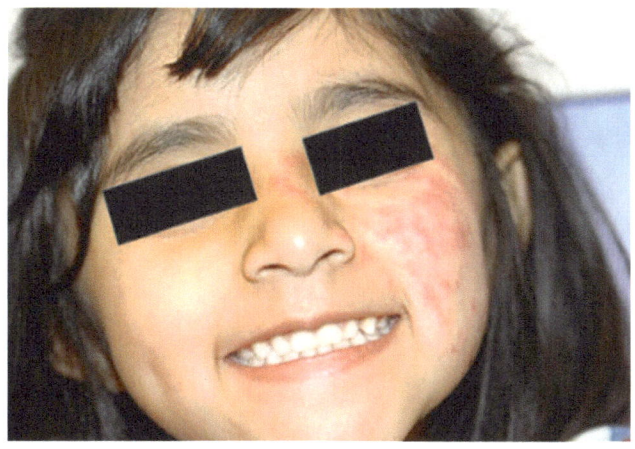

   (a) Tinea faciei
   (b) Atopic dermatitis
   (c) Sarcoidosis
   (d) Seborrheic dermatitis

27. **A 5-year-old child presents with perianal itching that is considerably worse at night. Your exam shows very mild erythema but several excoriations. What is the most accurate statement regarding the diagnosis?**
   (a) Infection is likely caused by group A streptococcus
   (b) Infection is likely caused by ingestion of pinworm eggs
   (c) Infection is always symptomatic
   (d) Recurrence of infection is rare

28. **This 4-year-old child presents with pain and itching to the perianal area. The mother states she has noticed blood-tinged stools as well. What is the most likely culprit?**

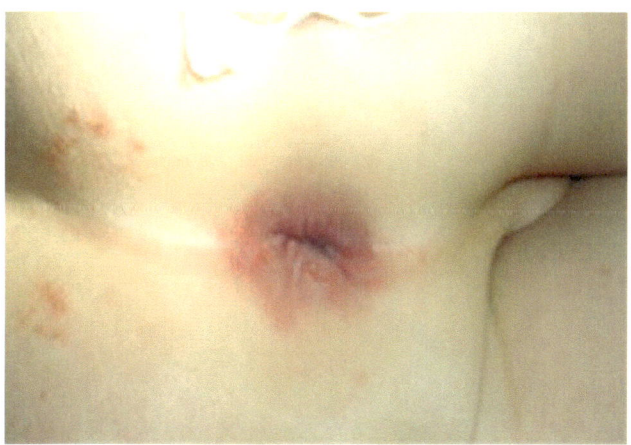

   (a) Infection caused by group A streptococcus
   (b) Infection caused by ingestion of pinworm eggs
   (c) Infection caused by Corynebacterium minutissimum
   (d) Irritation caused by irritant contact dermatitis

29. **A child presents with a low-grade fever and a rash to the lower legs accompanied by a burning sensation. On examination, there are purpuric macules that coalesce together but abruptly stop at the ankles. What is the most likely cause?**

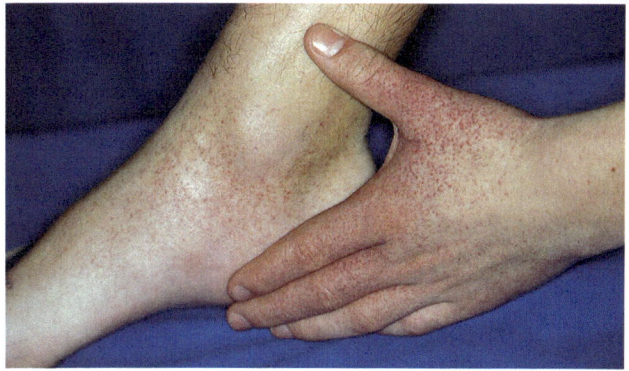

   (a) Group A beta-hemolytic streptococci
   (b) Varicella-zoster virus
   (c) Coxsackievirus
   (d) Parvovirus B19

30. **Purpuric macules and papules to lower extremities and buttocks are seen in this child with accompanying joint pain. What would you most likely see on direct immunofluorescence (DIF)?**

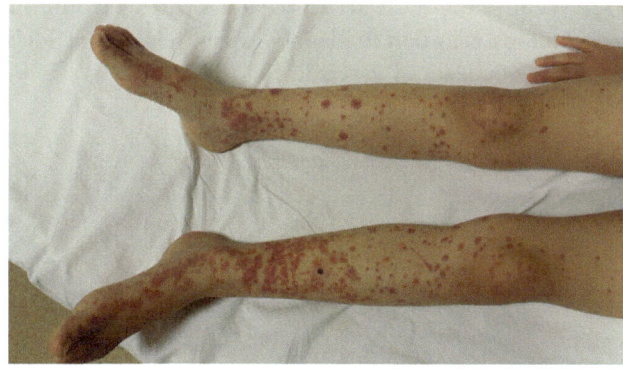

   (a) Negative DIF
   (b) Perivascular IgA
   (c) Perivascular IgG
   (d) Granular IgA deposits in papillary dermis

31. **Which of the following is the least likely association in a child with these erythematous scaly patches and plaques over the dorsal hand shown in the figure?**

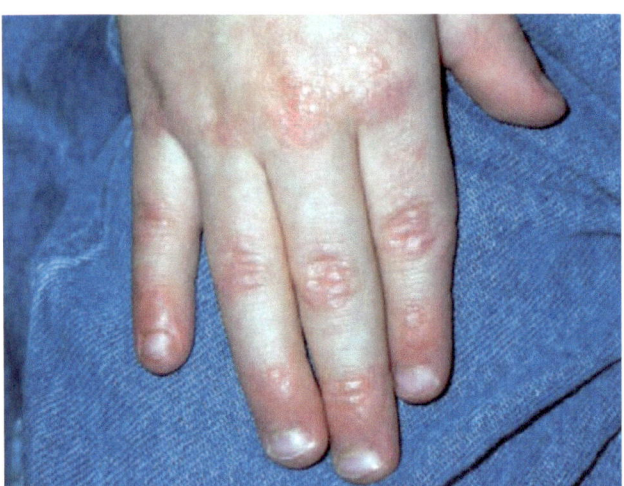

(a) Elevated creatine kinase
(b) Calcinosis involving elbows, knees, buttocks and areas of trauma
(c) Muscular deficit that is asymmetric and starts with distal muscle weakness
(d) Pulmonary manifestations including interstitial lung disease and respiratory muscle involvement

32. **What is the most accurate statement regarding the bullous eruption in this 4-year-old child that looks like a "cluster of jewels" ?**

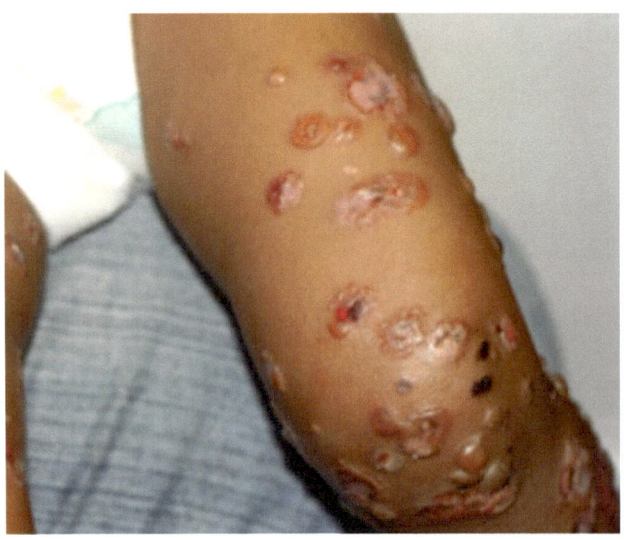

(a) The direct immunofluorescence (DIF) would show linear staining with IgA
(b) The DIF would show perivascular IgA
(c) The DIF would show intercellular IgA
(d) The DIF would be negative

33. **What is most likely the correct diagnosis for this child?**

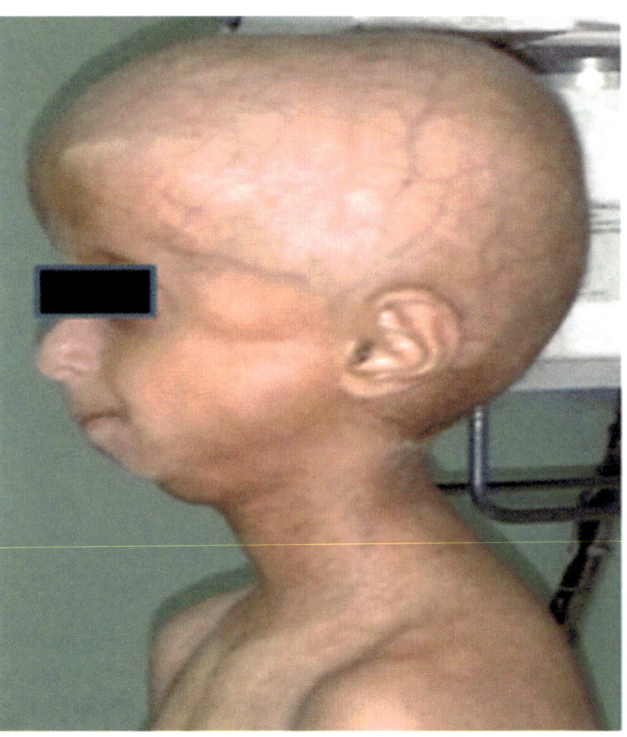

(a) Werner syndrome
(b) Progeria syndrome
(c) Hyper-IgE syndrome
(d) Wiskott-Aldrich syndrome

34. **Death in the above patient (question 33) will most likely occur due to which of the following?**

(a) Severe premature coronary atherosclerosis
(b) Bone marrow failure
(c) Gastrointestinal adenocarcinoma
(d) Thyroid follicular carcinoma

35. The abnormality seen in the patient's teeth in the figure is a feature seen in which of the following syndromes?

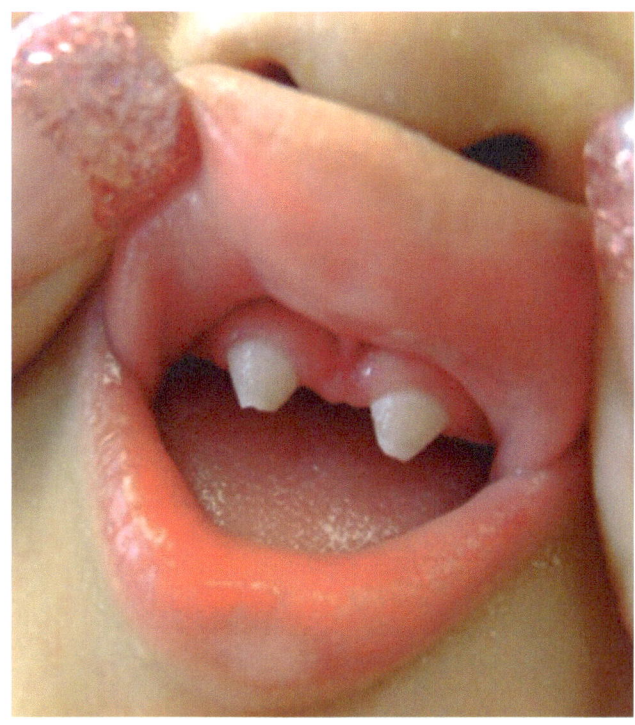

(a) Papillon-Lefèvre syndrome
(b) Anhidrotic ectodermal dysplasia
(c) Gardner syndrome
(d) Hyperimmunoglobulin E syndrome

36. What would be the best management option for the patient with the following presentation of painless bluish to purple nodules to the hands and feet along with the lesions pictured below (white arrows)?

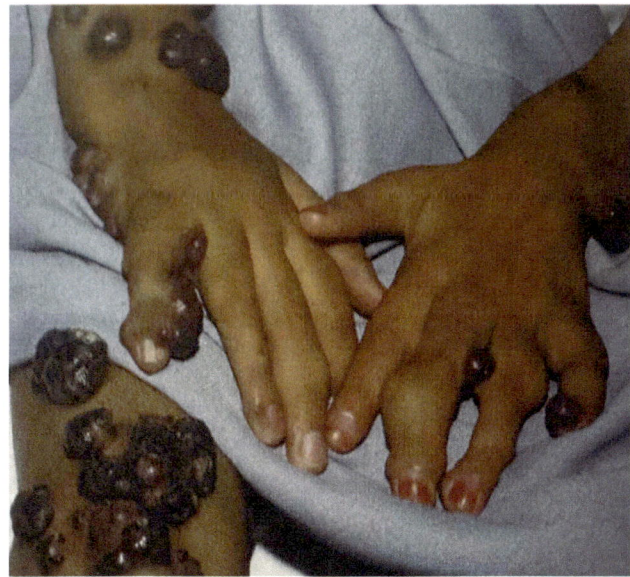

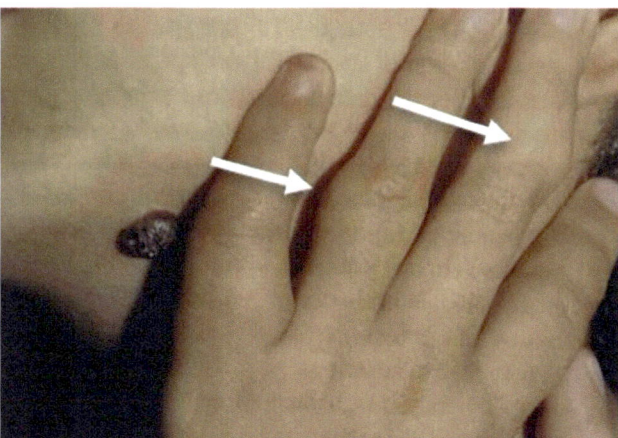

(a) Monitor endochondromas to discern if any malignant transformation to chondrosarcoma
(b) Send to a gastrointestinal (GI) physician for endoscopy to evaluate any GI venous malformations that may cause GI bleeding
(c) Monitor for potential intussusception and venous malformation in GI tract
(d) Monitor for any dyspnea from potential pulmonary arteriovenous malformations

37. A child presents with soft bluish nodules on his hands, painful especially at night, with increased sweating to the affected areas. Your biggest concern in this patient is which of the following?

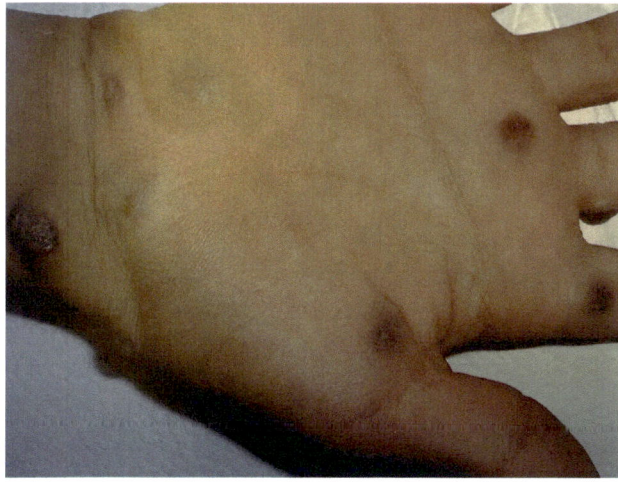

(a) Gastrointestinal (GI) adenocarcinoma
(b) Aortic coarctation
(c) Chondrosarcoma
(d) GI bleeding

38. Which is the least likely condition to see genital lentigines?
(a) Bannayan-Riley-Ruvalcaba syndrome
(b) Carney complex
(c) Laugier-Hunziker syndrome
(d) Peutz-Jeghers syndrome

39. **The pathology in the baby shown in the figure showing extensive bullae along with perioral exuberant granulation tissue will most likely have a defect in which of the following?**

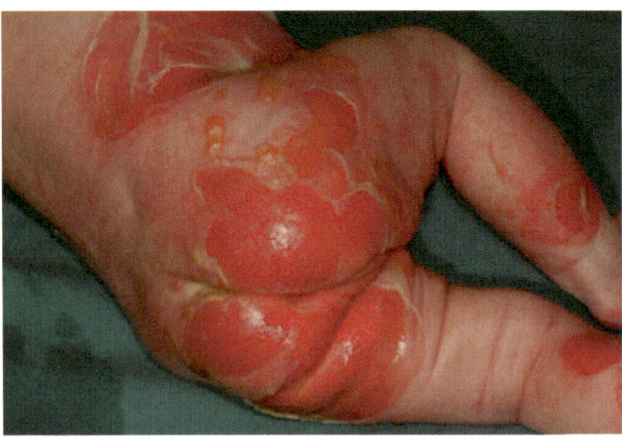

   (a) Laminin-332
   (b) K5, K14
   (c) Plectin
   (d) Type VII collagen

40. **This figure shows a 10-year-old boy's plantar feet. The patient complains of irritation often after recess and playing sports. Which of the following is the least accurate statement regarding this diagnosis?**

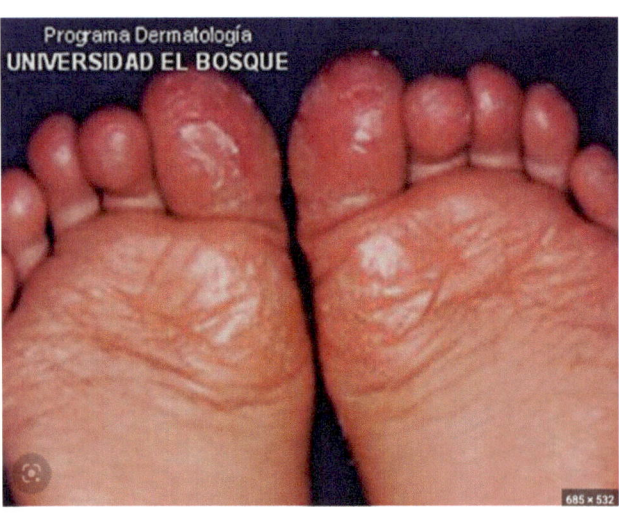

   (a) It is worsened by repetitive frictional movement and/or an occlusive effect
   (b) It typically affects both feet symmetrically
   (c) Treatment includes using tight-fitting shoes
   (d) This will often clear spontaneously in adolescence but can persist into adult life

Answer Key

1. a
2. e
3. c
4. a
5. b
6. a
7. e
8. c
9. a
10. b
11. c
12. d
13. a
14. d
15. b
16. a
17. e
18. a
19. c
20. d
21. e
22. a
23. a
24. e
25. a
26. a
27. b
28. a
29. d
30. b
31. c
32. a
33. b
34. a
35. b
36. a
37. d
38. d
39. a
40. c

Image Sources

2.1 Pope, E., Deodhare, N., Lara-Corrales, I. (2018). Neonate Dermatology. In: Smoller, B., Bagherani, N. (eds) Atlas of Dermatology, Dermatopathology and Venereology. Springer, Cham. https://link.springer.com/referenceworkentry/10.1007/978-3-319-45134-3_25-1#Fig6

2.3 Phung, T.L., Wright, T.S., Pourciau, C.Y., Smoller, B.R. (2017). Diseases of Collagen and Elastic Tissue. In: Pediatric Dermatopathology. Springer, Cham. https://doi.org/10.1007/978-3-319-44824-4_7

2.4 Tubbs RS, Oskouian RJ, Blount JP, Oakes WP. Occult Spinal Dysraphism, 2019. Springer, Cham. https://link.springer.com/chapter/10.1007/978-3-030-10994-3_4

2.5 Phung TL, Wright TS, Pourciau, CY, Smoller BR. Pediatric Dermatopathology, Springer, Cham 2017.

2.6 Phung, T.L., Wright, T.S., Pourciau, C.Y., Smoller, B.R. (2017). Disorders of Pigmentation. In: Pediatric Dermatopathology. Springer, Cham. https://doi.org/10.1007/978-3-319-44824-4_17

2.7 Phung, T.L., Wright, T.S., Pourciau, C.Y., Smoller, B.R. (2017). Disorders of Pigmentation. In: Pediatric Dermatopathology. Springer, Cham. https://doi.org/10.1007/978-3-319-44824-4_17

2.8 Phung, T.L., Wright, T.S., Pourciau, C.Y., Smoller, B.R. (2017). Interface Dermatoses. In: Pediatric Dermatopathology. Springer, Cham. https://doi.org/10.1007/978-3-319-44824-4_4

2.9 Phung, T.L., Wright, T.S., Pourciau, C.Y., Smoller, B.R. (2017). Nutritional Disorders. In: Pediatric Dermatopathology. Springer, Cham. https://doi.org/10.1007/978-3-319-44824-4_15

2.10 Phung, T.L., Wright, T.S., Pourciau, C.Y., Smoller, B.R. (2017). Vascular Anomalies. In: Pediatric Dermatopathology. Springer, Cham. https://doi.org/10.1007/978-3-319-44824-4_21

2.11 Schneider, M. (2022). Vascular Tumours (Haemangiomas). In: Panteliadis, C.P., Benjamin, R., Hagel, C. (eds) Neurocutaneous Disorders. Springer, Cham. https://doi.org/10.1007/978-3-030-87893-1_25

2.13 Phung, T.L., Wright, T.S., Pourciau, C.Y., Smoller, B.R. (2017). Benign Hamartomatous Proliferations. In: Pediatric Dermatopathology. Springer, Cham. https://doi.org/10.1007/978-3-319-44824-4_29

2.14 Al-Salem, A.H. (2020). Dermoid Cysts. In: Atlas of Pediatric Surgery. Springer, Cham. https://doi.org/10.1007/978-3-030-29211-9_4

2.15 Phung, T.L., Wright, T.S., Pourciau, C.Y., Smoller, B.R. (2017). Fibrous Proliferations. In: Pediatric Dermatopathology. Springer, Cham. https://doi.org/10.1007/978-3-319-44824-4_25

2.16 Phung, T.L., Wright, T.S., Pourciau, C.Y., Smoller, B.R. (2017). Hematopoietic Proliferations. In: Pediatric Dermatopathology. Springer, Cham. https://doi.org/10.1007/978-3-319-44824-4_22

2.18 Phung, T.L., Wright, T.S., Pourciau, C.Y., Smoller, B.R. (2017). Hematopoietic Proliferations. In: Pediatric Dermatopathology. Springer, Cham. https://doi.org/10.1007/978-3-319-44824-4_22

2.19 Requena, L., Sangüeza, O. Pilomatricoma. In: Cutaneous Adnexal Neoplasms. Cham, Switzerland: Springer; 2017. pp 645–69. https://doi.org/10.1007/978-3-319-45704-8_52

2.20 Phung, T.L., Wright, T.S., Pourciau, C.Y., Smoller, B.R. (2017). Fibrous Proliferations. In: Pediatric Dermatopathology. Springer, Cham. https://doi.org/10.1007/978-3-319-44824-4_25

2.21 Phung, T.L., Wright, T.S., Pourciau, C.Y., Smoller, B.R. (2017). Tumors of the Cutaneous Appendages and the Epidermis. In: Pediatric Dermatopathology. Springer, Cham. https://doi.org/10.1007/978-3-319-44824-4_24

2.22 Phung, T.L., Wright, T.S., Pourciau, C.Y., Smoller, B.R. (2017). Keratinous Cysts and Hamartomas. In: Pediatric Dermatopathology. Springer, Cham. https://doi.org/10.1007/978-3-319-44824-4_23

2.23 Lacarrubba, F., Verzì, A.E., Nasca, M.R., Micali, G. (2018). Congenital Triangular Alopecia. In: Micali, G., Lacarrubba, F., Stinco, G., Argenziano, G., Neri, I. (eds) Atlas of Pediatric Dermatoscopy. Springer, Cham. pp 163–167. https://doi.org/10.1007/978-3-319-71168-3_23

2.24 Bhandari, B., Singh, R., Kumar, M. et al. Acute Hemorrhagic Edema of Infancy. Indian J Pediatr 85, 245–246 (2018). https://link.springer.com/article/10.1007/s12098-017-2463-5

2.25 Pilania, R.K., Singh, S. (2020). Kawasaki Disease. In: Cimaz, R. (eds) Periodic and Non-Periodic Fevers. Rare Diseases of the Immune System. Springer, Cham. pp 45–63. https://doi.org/10.1007/978-3-030-19055-2_4

2.26 Phung, T.L., Wright, T.S., Pourciau, C.Y., Smoller, B.R. (2017). Fungal Diseases. In: Pediatric Dermatopathology. Springer, Cham. https://doi.org/10.1007/978-3-319-44824-4_13

2.28 Jongen, J., Eberstein, A., Peleikis, HG. et al. Perianal Streptococcal Dermatitis: An Important Differential Diagnosis in Pediatric Patients. Dis Colon Rectum 51, 584–587 (2008). https://doi.org/10.1007/s10350-008-9237-0

2.29 Fölster-Holst, R. (2022). Other Viral Infections of the Skin. In: Plewig, G., French, L., Ruzicka, T., Kaufmann, R., Hertl, M. (eds) Braun-Falco's Dermatology. Springer, Berlin, Heidelberg. https://doi.org/10.1007/978-3-662-63709-8_10

2.30 Yılmaz, N., Yüksel, S., Becerir, T. et al. Myocarditis and intracardiac thrombus due to Henoch-Schönlein purpura: case report and literature review. Clin Rheumatol 40, 1635–1644 (2021). https://doi.org/10.1007/s10067-020-05317-8

2.31 Walling, H.W., Gerami, P. & Sontheimer, R.D. Juvenile-Onset Clinically Amyopathic Dermatomyositis. Pediatr-Drugs 12, 23–34 (2010). https://doi.org/10.2165/10899380-000000000-00000

2.32 Phung, T.L., Wright, T.S., Pourciau, C.Y., Smoller, B.R. (2017). Vesiculobullous Diseases. In: Pediatric Dermatopathology. Springer, Cham. https://doi.org/10.1007/978-3-319-44824-4_3

2.33 Reprint from Chawla, G.S., Agrawal, P.M. & Dhok, A. Progeria: an extremely unusual disorder. Skeletal Radiol 46, 1149–1153 (2017). https://doi.org/10.1007/s00256-017-2673-y

2.35 Phung, T.L., Wright, T.S., Pourciau, C.Y., Smoller, B.R. (2017). Diseases of the Hair and Nails. In: Pediatric Dermatopathology. Springer, Cham. https://doi.org/10.1007/978-3-319-44824-4_18

2.36 Baykal, C., Yazganoğlu, K.D. (2014). Vascular Anomalies. In: Clinical Atlas of Skin Tumors. Springer, Berlin, Heidelberg, 169–230. https://doi.org/10.1007/978-3-642-40938-7_6

2.37 Reprint from Baykal C, Yazganoglu KD. Clinical Atlas of Skin Tumors. Springer Heidelburg 2014.

2.39 Laimer, M., Bauer, J.W., Hintner, H. (2015). Generalized Severe Junctional Epidermolysis Bullosa. In: Murrell, D. (eds) Blistering Diseases. Springer, Berlin, Heidelberg. https://doi.org/10.1007/978-3-662-45698-9_36

2.40 Motta A, González LF, García G, Guzmán J, Prada L, Herrera H. et al. (2022). Papulosquamous and Eczematous Dermatoses: Dermatitis. In: Atlas of Dermatology. Springer, Cham. https://doi.org/10.1007/978-3-030-84107-2_1

1. The most likely diagnosis in this patient with abdominal pain, oral lesions, and isolated scrotal swelling is:

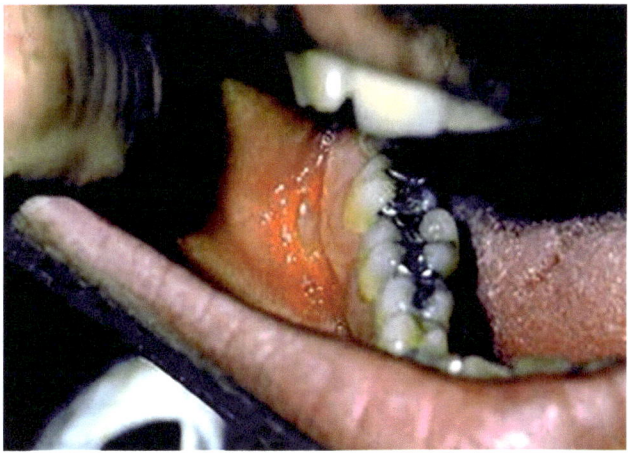

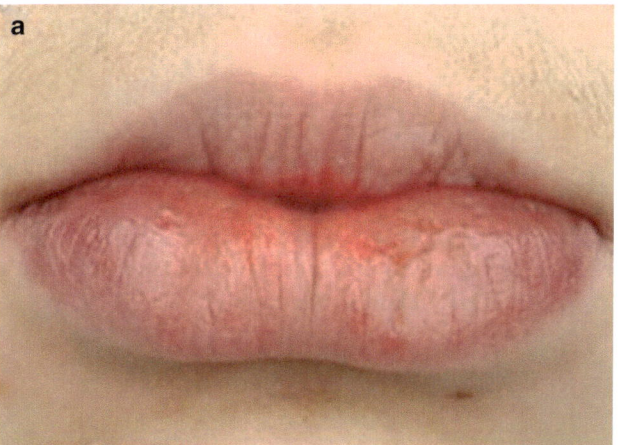

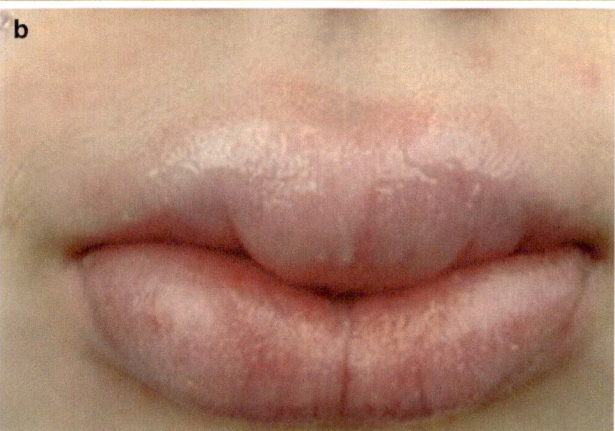

   (a) Crohn's disease
   (b) Ulcerative colitis
   (c) Pemphigus vulgaris
   (d) Lichen planus
   (e) Oral white sponge nevus

2. A 13-year-old female presented with recurrent and persistent swelling of her lower lip but denied any symptoms of intestinal disease such as abdominal pain, diarrhea, or weight loss. No further workup was performed. Topical clobetasol was initiated but with little effect. A few months later the patient developed increased swelling to her upper lip along with abdominal pain, altered bowel habits and weight loss. Of note, she had no changes to her tongue and no evidence facial nerve paralysis on exam. What is the most likely diagnosis?

   (a) Cheilitis granulomatosa as an extraintestinal manifestation of ulcerative colitis
   (b) Cheilitis granulomatosa (or granulomatous cheilitis) as an extraintestinal manifestation of Crohn's disease
   (c) Cheilitis glandularis as a manifestation of hepatitis C
   (d) Cheilitis glandularis as manifestation of multiple endocrine neoplasia (MEN) 2B
   (e) Melkersson-Rosenthal syndrome

3. **Cutaneous manifestations of inflammatory bowel disease (IBD) tend to improve with adequate treatment of the underlying bowel disease.**

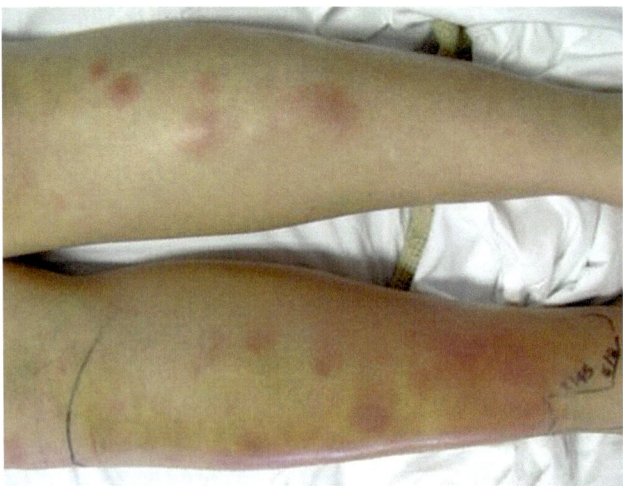

   (a) True
   (b) False

4. **Erythema nodosum is not typically associated with which of the following conditions?**

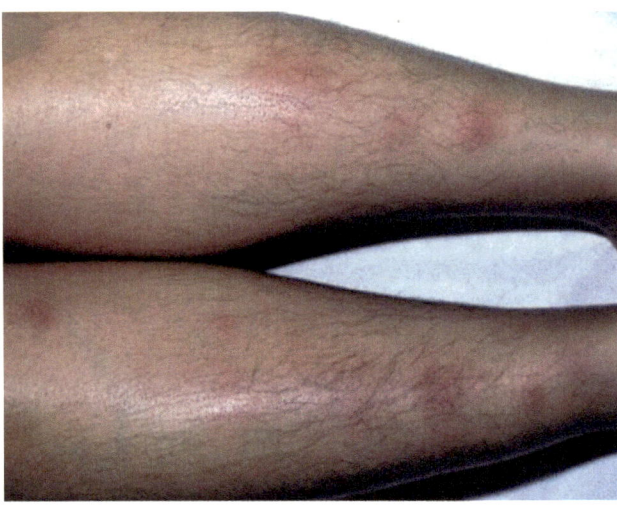

   (a) Strep infection
   (b) Sarcoidosis
   (c) Birth control pill use
   (d) Oral sulfonamide use
   (e) Crohn's disease
   (f) Diabetes mellitus

5. **This 22-year-old male with no past medical history has recurrent red-brown firm papulonodules on his upper arms that are in different stages for the past 1 year that regress on their own and then recur. The areas are not tender and there is no discharge or fluctuance. Prior lesions are flat but still discolored. He has no other symptoms or cutaneous lesions elsewhere. The most likely diagnosis is:**

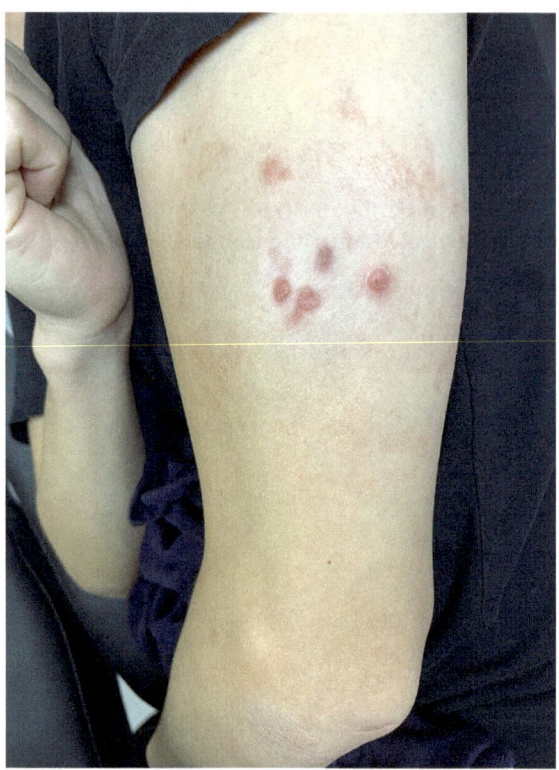

   (a) Mycosis fungoides
   (b) Lymphomatoid papulosis
   (c) Sweet syndrome
   (d) Polymorphous light eruption

6. **Erythema nodosum is considered a good prognostic sign for sarcoidosis.**
   (a) True
   (b) False

7. **A patient presents with a painful rash on her face for the past 3 weeks. She feels well overall except for facial tenderness. She denies any fever, muscle aches or joint pain. What is the best initial treatment to acutely improve her symptoms?**

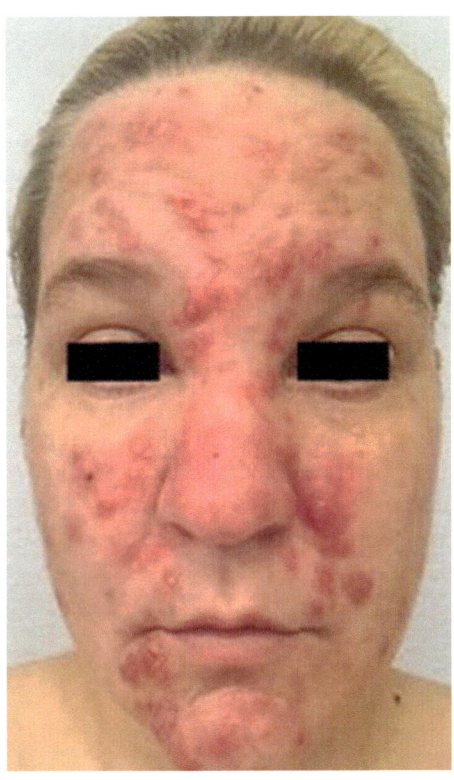

   (a) Doxycycline 100 mg twice daily
   (b) Prednisone 40 mg once daily
   (c) Isotretinoin 40 mg once daily
   (d) Spironolactone 100 mg once daily

8. **The percentage of patients with psoriasis who already have psoriatic arthritis or will have psoriatic arthritis in the future is approximately:**
   (a) 20–30%
   (b) 5–10%
   (c) 50–75%
   (d) <1%

9. **Which of the following interleukins specifically plays a central role in the pathogenesis of pustular psoriasis?**
   (a) IL-36
   (b) IL-4
   (c) IL-13
   (d) IL-23

10. **The risk of developing cutaneous squamous cell carcinoma in longstanding vulvar lichen sclerosus et atrophicus is approximately what percent?**

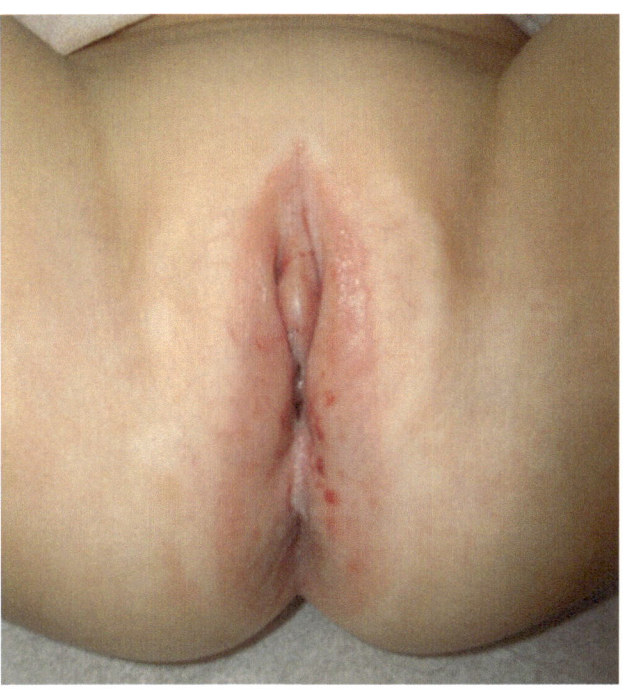

   (a) 20%
   (b) 5%
   (c) 75%
   (d) <1%

11. **A 39-year-old overweight female presents with a 5-month history of a rash on her lower legs that is asymptomatic but slowly expanding. She has no medical problems and is not on any medications. She denies any similar rashes in the past or other areas. What is the most likely diagnosis?**

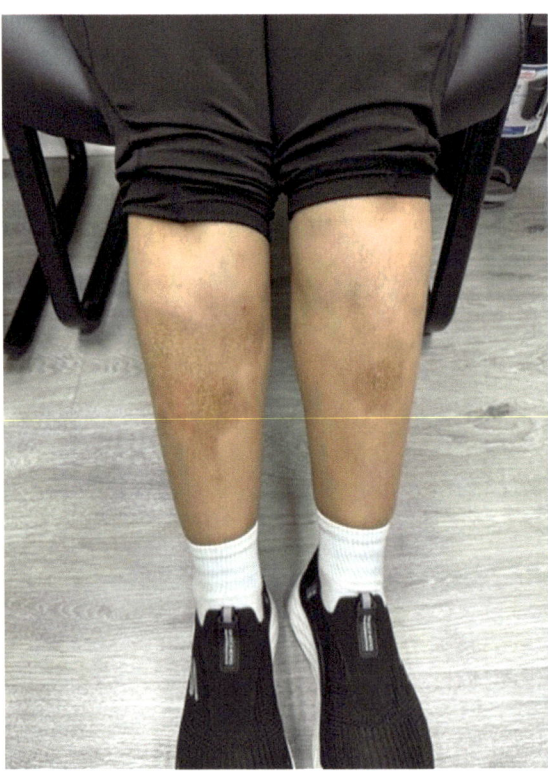

(a) Necrobiosis lipoidica
(b) Erythema induratum
(c) Erythema nodosum
(d) Granuloma annulare

12. **Factors that contribute to acne inversa (hidradenitis suppurativa) include all of the following except:**
    (a) Weight gain
    (b) Tobacco use
    (c) Insulin resistance
    (d) Excess sweating
    (e) Tight fitting clothing
    (f) Stress
    (g) Low glycemic index diet

13. **The best treatment for an overweight patient with hidradenitis suppurativa, androgenetic alopecia, and increased terminal hairs to her chin and sideburn areas would be:**
    (a) Oral retinoid due to follicular occlusion
    (b) Oral metformin with possible oral contraceptive pill and spironolactone for likely metabolic dysfunction
    (c) Oral antibiotic for the dysbiosis seen in hidradenitis suppurativa
    (d) Exercise, weight loss, and loose-fitting clothing as monotherapy to reduce friction/irritation to affected areas

14. **A patient with Roux-en-Y gastric bypass, history of alcohol use, and end-stage liver disease presents with a painful skin eruption and malaise for 3 weeks. The rash started around her mouth but now has spread to her feet, thigh, buttocks, perianal area, and elbows. She tried a topical steroid course (triamcinolone 0.1% ointment twice daily for 2 weeks) but the rash did not improve. What is the most likely diagnosis?**

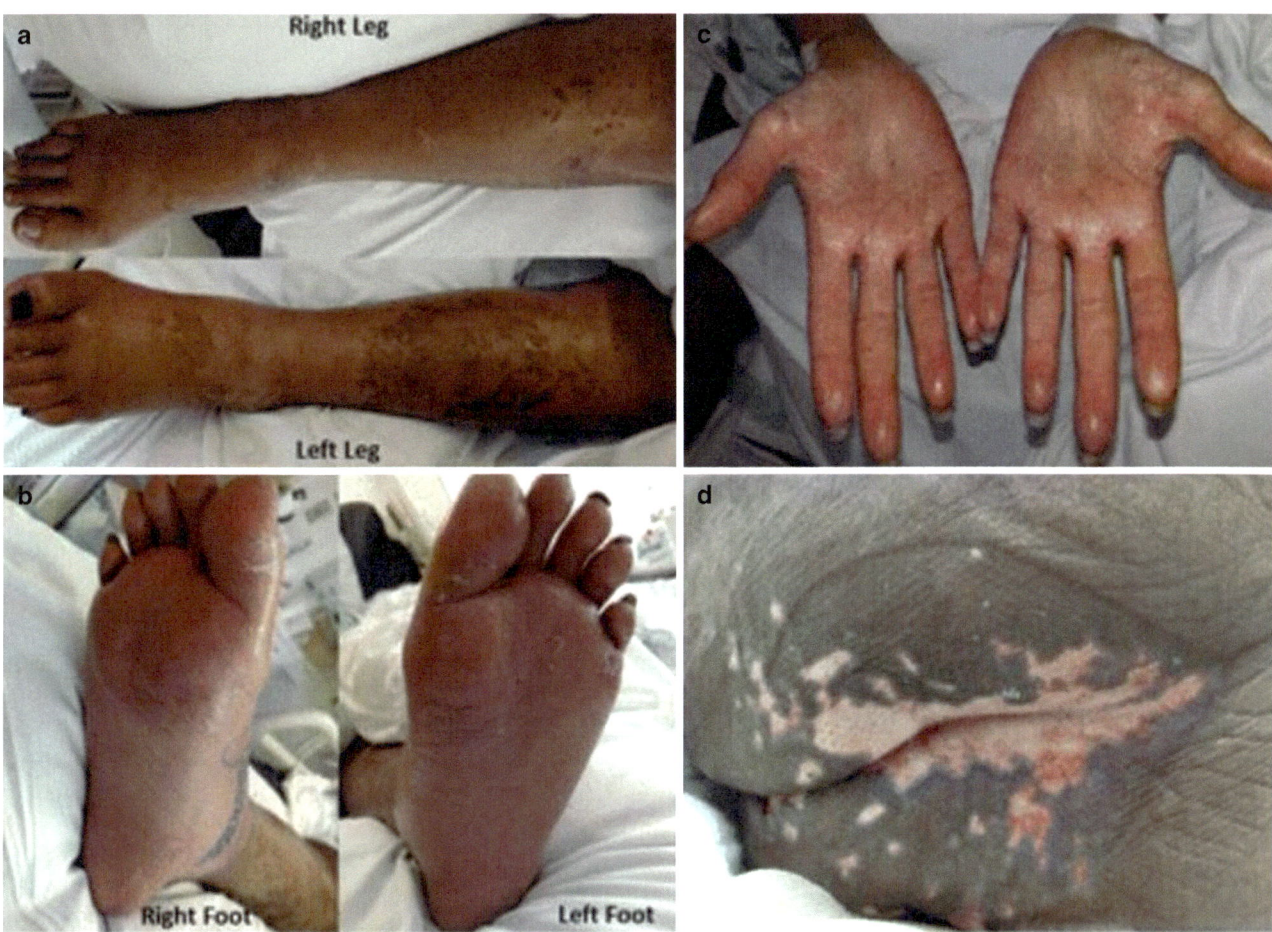

(a) Acquired acrodermatitis enteropathica

(b) Necrolytic migratory erythema

(c) Pellagra

(d) Necrolytic acral erythema

15. **A 32-year-old patient presents with discoloration and thickening to the neck that has been present for several years. Lab work would most likely show which of the following to be abnormally elevated?**

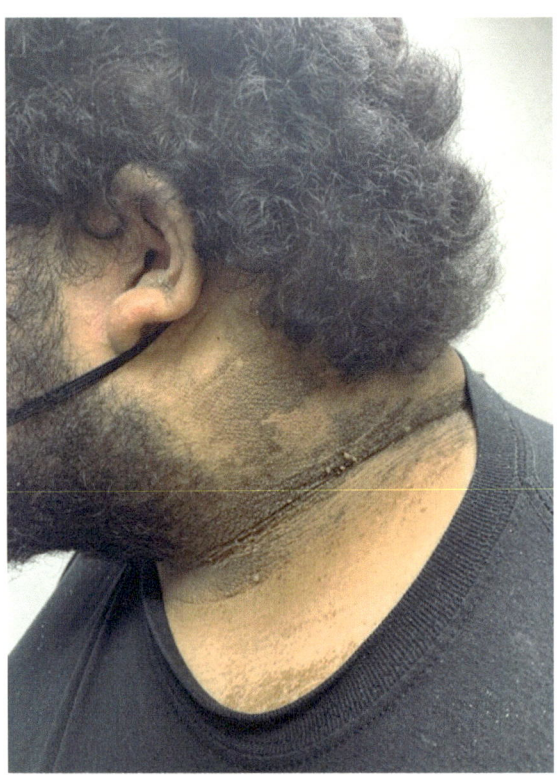

   (a) Total and free testosterone
   (b) Dehydroepiandrosterone (DHEA) sulfate
   (c) Luteinizing hormone (LH)
   (d) Fasting insulin

16. **A 30-year-old female presents with acne, irregular menses, increased facial hair growth to the upper cutaneous lip, and alopecia involving the centroparietal scalp for the past 10 years. Which of the following lab tests will most likely NOT be elevated in this patient?**

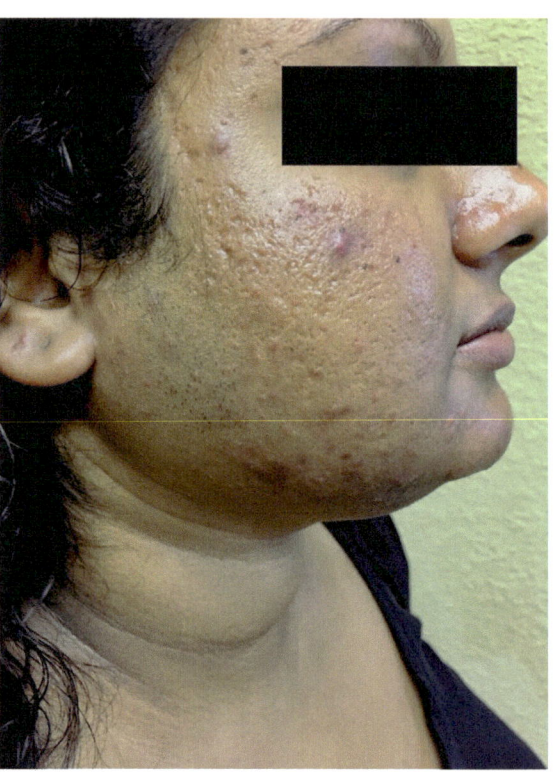

   (a) Free testosterone
   (b) Dehydroepiandrosterone (DHEA) sulfate
   (c) Androstenedione
   (d) Sex-hormone binding globulin
   (e) Fasting insulin

17. **Which statement is the most accurate regarding the diagnosis of lichen planus (LP)?**
   (a) Cutaneous lichen planus often clears spontaneously in approximately 4–5 months
   (b) Linear LP appears to be more common in adults than children
   (c) Drug-induced LP can be seen with thiazide diuretics, non-steroidal anti-inflammatory drugs (NSAIDs), angiotensin-converting enzyme inhibitors (ACEIs) and antimalarials
   (d) Approximately, 20% of patients with cutaneous LP have concomitant hepatitis C

18. **Treatment with an oral contraceptive pill (combination of estrogen/progestin) can be helpful in women with polycystic ovarian syndrome (PCOS) due to the following?**
    (a) It increases the production of sex hormonal binding globulin (SHBG) which leads to a decrease in free testosterone
    (b) It decreases the production of SHBG and leads to a decrease in total testosterone, but not free testosterone
    (c) It increases the production of SHBG and leads to an increase in total testosterone
    (d) It decreases the production of SHBG and leads to a decrease in free testosterone

19. **This 21-year-old female presents with hair loss that she states started when she was 13 years old. She was seen by her pediatrician at that time and was told there was no treatment and the cause of her hair loss was unclear. She is not sure if she had blood work back then. The hair loss has progressively gotten worse and she denies any itching, scaling or pain to the area. Patient overall feels well and has no medical problems. She denies any irregularity of her menses, no hirsutism or acne. She is on no medications. What is the next step?**

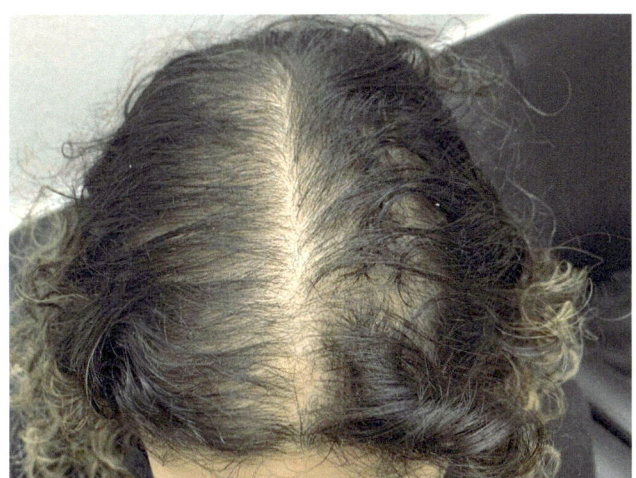

    (a) Check blood work including androgen levels for potential polycystic ovarian syndrome and 17-hydroxyprogesterone for possible non-classic congenital adrenal hyperplasia (NCAH)
    (b) Check thyroid function tests and anti-thyroglobulin and anti-thyroid peroxidase antibodies for autoimmune thyroid dysfunction
    (c) Check cortisol level for underlying Cushing syndrome
    (d) Check fasting insulin level for underlying insulinoma
    (e) Do not check any as the patient has androgenetic alopecia and her lab findings will be within normal limits

20. **This patient with small, monomorphic papules to the forehead, loss of eyebrow hair and recession to frontal and temporal hairline with mild perifollicular scale on dermoscopic exam most likely has:**

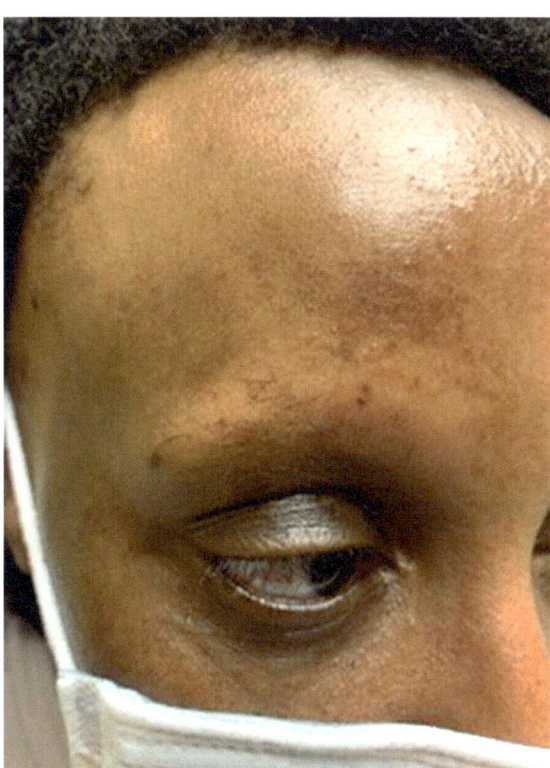

    (a) Central centrifugal cicatricial alopecia (CCCA)
    (b) Lichen planopilaris (LPP)
    (c) Frontal fibrosing alopecia (FFA)
    (d) Follicular mucinosis
    (e) Follicular mycosis fungoides

21. **A 55-year-old woman presents with a 3-month history of intense itching to her scalp and hair loss. A** dermoscopic image is provided as well. The most likely diagnosis is:

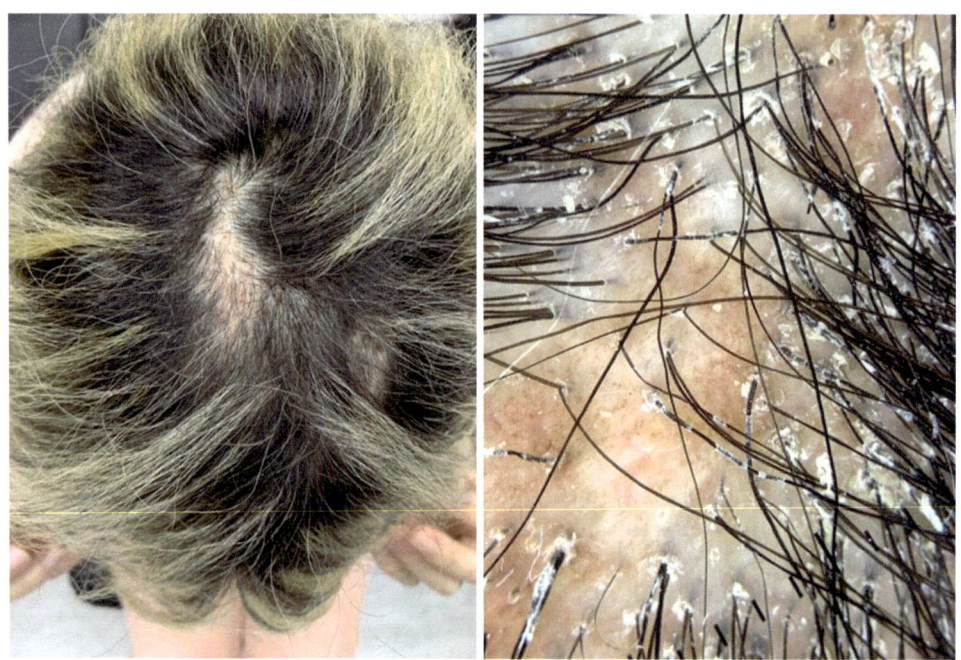

(a) Central centrifugal cicatricial alopecia (CCCA)
(b) Lichen planopilaris (LPP)
(c) Frontal fibrosing alopecia (FFA)
(d) Follicular mucinosis
(e) Follicular mycosis fungoides

22. **A 55-year-old female presents with a 15-year history of hair loss to the areas shown in the figure. She denies any pain, tingling, scaling or tenderness to the affected areas. What is the most likely diagnosis?**

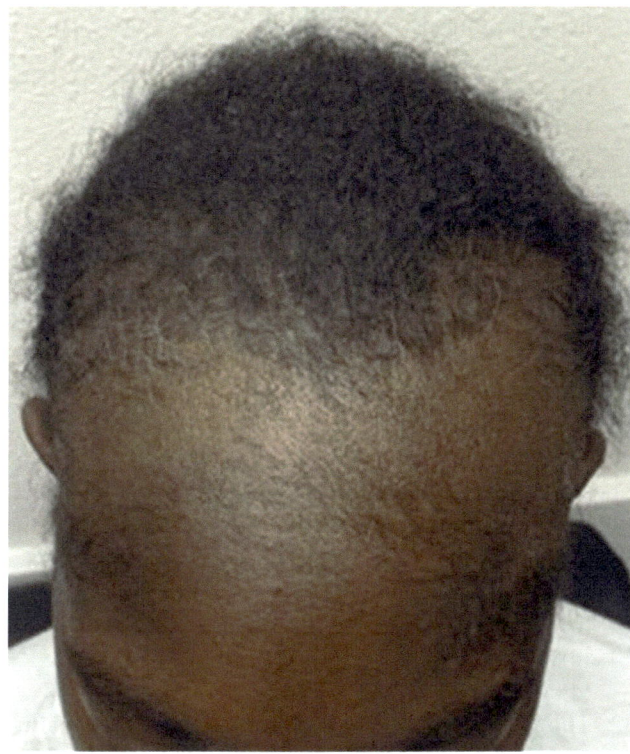

 (a) Central centrifugal cicatricial alopecia (CCCA)
 (b) Lichen planopilaris (LPP)
 (c) Frontal fibrosing alopecia (FFA)
 (d) Traction alopecia
 (e) Androgenetic alopecia

23. **What are dermoscopic signs of active, ongoing inflammation in alopecia areata?**
 (a) Exclamation mark hairs and black dots
 (b) Yellow dots
 (c) Bent hairs
 (d) Corkscrew hairs

24. **The below listed changes are related to a defect in the nail matrix except:**
 (a) Pitting
 (b) Onychodystrophy
 (c) Leukonychia
 (d) Oil spots

25. **Superficial punctate depressions in the nail plate as seen in the center of the nail in the figure are due to an abnormality in the:**

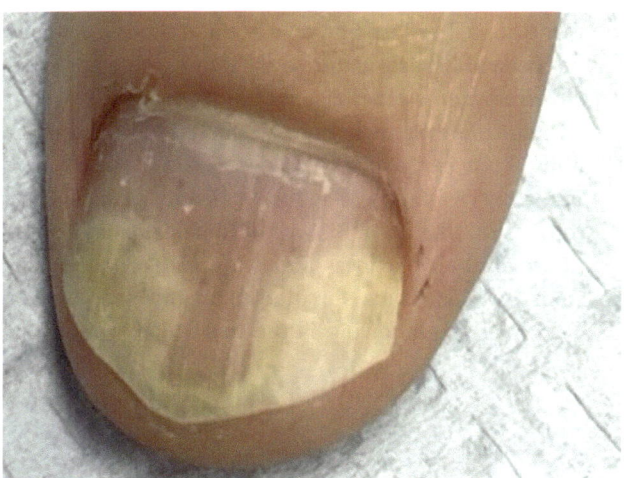

 (a) Nail bed
 (b) Proximal nail matrix
 (c) Distal matrix

26. **A 25-year-old female presents with discoloration to her wrists for 4 weeks. She states she noticed the discoloration the day after she came home from work. The patient is a bartender and was making drinks the night before for customers. On further questioning, the patient states she was wearing short gloves on her hands to protect her new manicure. What is the most likely culprit for the patient's discoloration?**

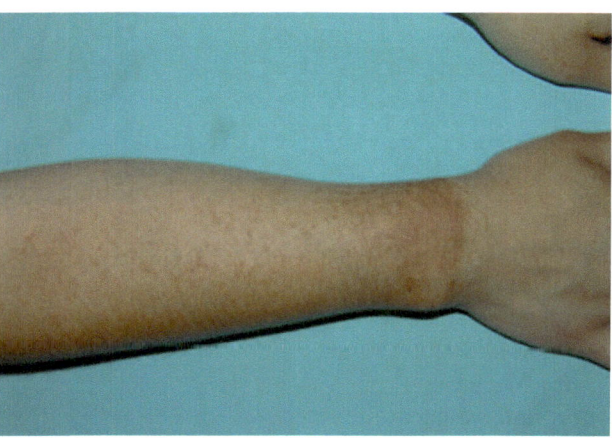

 (a) Lime juice
 (b) Cranberry juice
 (c) Ginger ale
 (d) Plum juice

27. A 77-year-old female presents with a 3-month history of a painful and itchy rash to her face for the past 3 months. She states it started when she was outdoors mid-day for 6 h without sunscreen, and when she came home her face felt very hot and tender. She has not been able to sleep due to the itching. She has tried clotrimazole-betamethasone dipropionate cream without improvement and she started topical terbinafine from her primary doctor but she thinks that made the rash worse. She has no history of sensitivity to the sun. She has a history of hypertension, hyperlipidemia and dizziness and is on different medications for this which she started in the past 1 year. Which of the following is the most likely culprit of her rash?

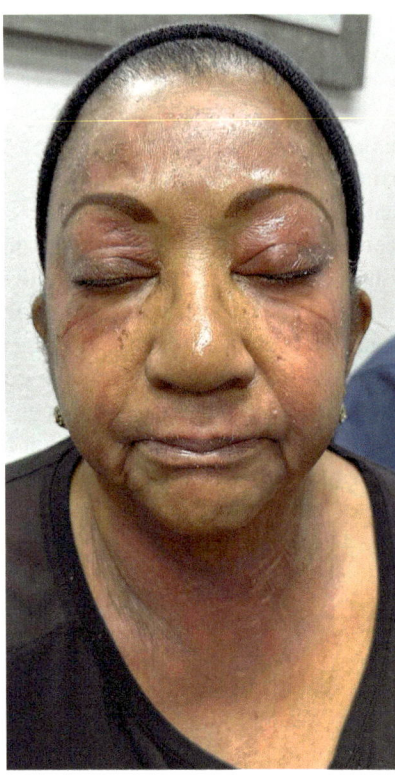

    (a) Metoprolol
    (b) Hydrochlorothiazide
    (c) Meclizine
    (d) Atorvastatin

28. **Purpuric contact dermatitis is most likely due to:**
    (a) Ethylene urea melamine formaldehyde
    (b) Methyl methacrylate
    (c) Mercaptobenzothiazole
    (d) Colophony
    (e) Cocamidopropyl betaine

29. A 25-year-old dental assistant presents with burning and tingling to her fingers for several months. She states at her job she manages daily adhesives and composite resins but always wears vinyl gloves while handling these substances. The most likely culprit of her symptoms is:
    (a) Ethylene urea melamine formaldehyde
    (b) Methyl methacrylate
    (c) Mercaptobenzothiazole
    (d) Colophony
    (e) Cocamidopropyl betaine

30. **Oral ingestion of the antihistamine hydroxyzine can be linked to exacerbation of an underlying contact dermatitis in patients with a sensitivity to which of the following?**
    (a) Ethylenediamine
    (b) Urushiol
    (c) Cocamidopropyl betaine
    (d) Neomycin sulfate

31. **The best way to differentiate acquired angioedema from hereditary angioedema is to check which of the following lab tests?**
    (a) C1q level
    (b) C1-inhibitor level
    (c) C1-inhibitor function
    (d) C4 level

32. **The following patient comes in for redness, itching and scaling around his lips for the past 2 days. He states he went to a fruit farm and tried various fruits and vegetables 3 days earlier. He does not have a rash on his chin or neck. He has no blisters or discoloration. Which is the most likely culprit?**

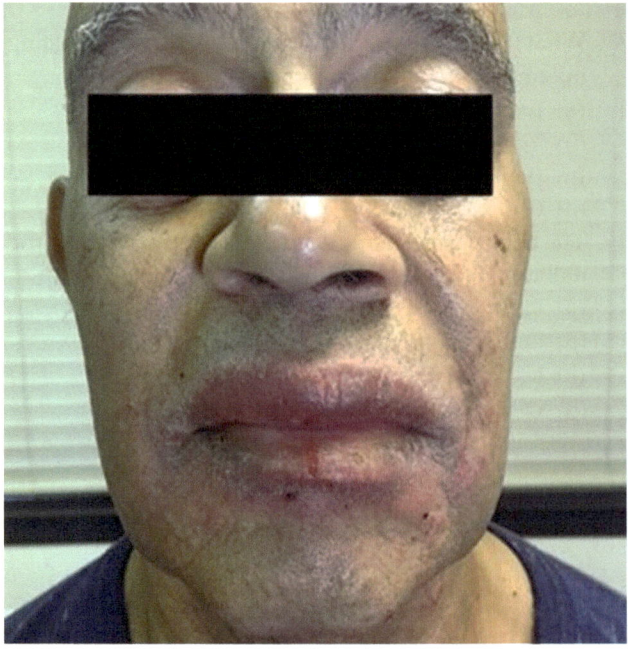

(a) Mango

(b) Celery

(c) Fig

(d) Lime

33. **Which of the following statements is not correct about the allergen urushiol?**

(a) The sap from the injured leaves, stems, and berries from the Anacardiaceae family (poison ivy, oak, and sumac) contains an oily resin called urushiol

(b) Fluid from ruptured vesicles will spread the eruption but the antigen retained on skin, clothing or fingernails will not result in spreading of the rash

(c) Once the immune system is triggered by penetration of the oily resin, washing the skin will not be helpful, so it is important to thoroughly wash the skin as soon as possible after the initial exposure (ideally within 20 min)

(d) Urushiol has cross-reactivity with other related plants such as the Japanese lacquer tree, mango rinds (peel, not pulp), cashew shell oil and gingko leaves

34. **A patient presents with itchy small blisters on her right ear lobe for the past 1 month and has noticed a new lesion on the superior aspect of her helix. She was given mupirocin ointment twice daily for 2 weeks with no improvement and a bacterial culture came back negative. She denies wearing any earrings and has not put anything to her ears that might cause a rash that she knows of. She has no history of similar reactions to her ear. The clinical appearance is shown in the picture, and her biopsy showed a subepidermal blister with eosinophils. Direct immunofluorescence (DIF) from perilesional skin is also shown. What is the most likely diagnosis in this patient?**

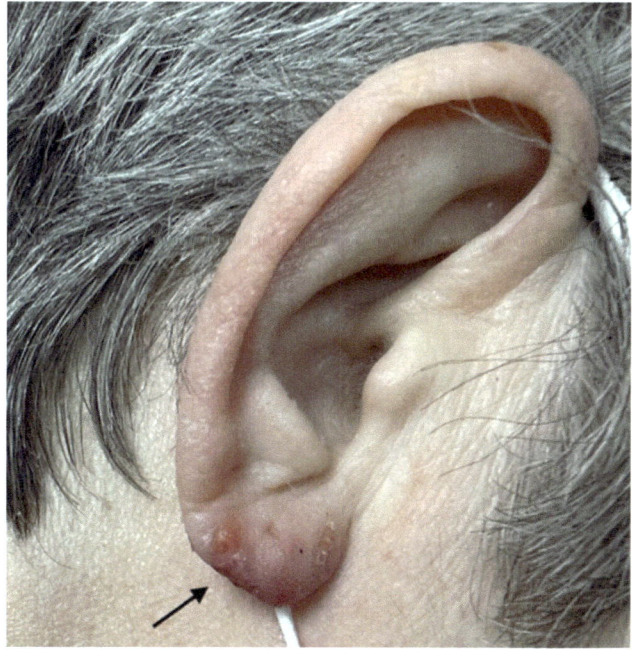

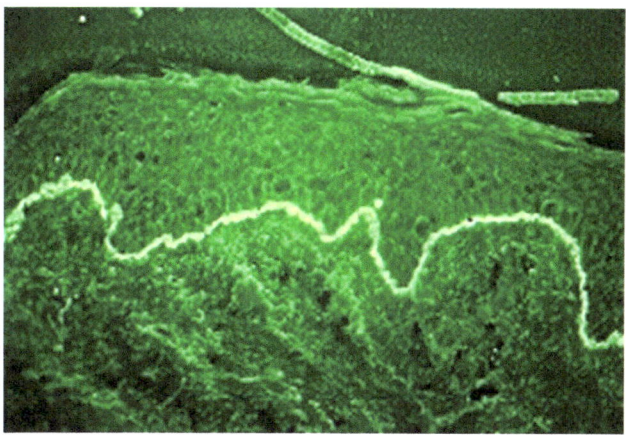

(a) Pemphigus vulgaris

(b) Paraneoplastic pemphigus

(c) Bullous pemphigoid

(d) Bullous systemic lupus erythematosus

(e) Porphyria cutanea tarda

35. **Direct immunofluorescence showing linear and intercellular IgG and C3 is most likely associated with:**

(a) Pemphigus vulgaris

(b) Bullous pemphigoid

(c) Dermatitis herpetiformis

(d) Paraneoplastic pemphigus

36. **Drug-induced pemphigus is mostly likely associated with which of the following drugs:**

(a) Captopril

(b) Trimethoprim/sulfamethoxazole

(c) Isoniazid

(d) Minocycline

37. **Which of the following paraneoplastic skin findings with likely associated cancer is NOT accurate?**

(a) Periorbital pinch purpura—primary systemic amyloidosis

(b) Necrolytic migratory erythema—pancreatic carcinoma

(c) Sweet syndrome—acute myelogenous leukemia

(d) Generalized pruritus—Hodgkin's lymphoma

(e) Psoriasiform plaques to the ear helices and nose—aerodigestive cancer

(f) Erythema nodosum—lung cancer

38. **A thin patient with no history of diabetes presents with new-onset asymptomatic rugose, velvety, white thickening of his hands along with accentuated dermatoglyphics and new-onset darkening and velvety thickening of his neck folds and axillae. What would you be most concerned about?**

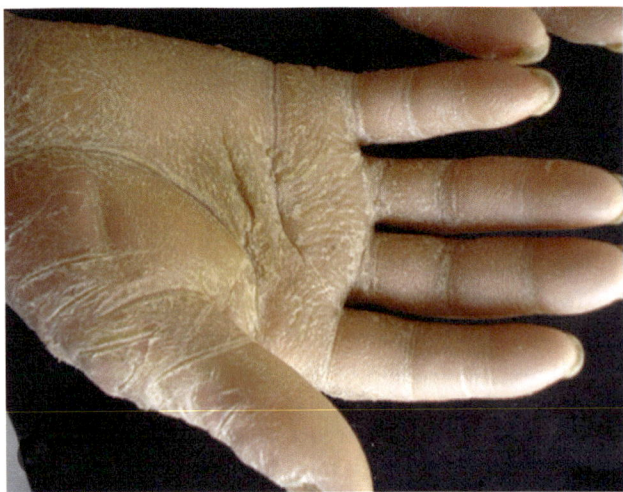

   (a) Underlying restrictive cardiomyopathy in systemic amyloidosis
   (b) Underlying gastrointestinal or lung cancer
   (c) Interstitial lung disease in anti-synthetase syndrome
   (d) Underlying lymphoproliferative disease

39. **What benign conditions may be associated with paraneoplastic pemphigus?**
   (a) Lymphoproliferative disorder with lymph node enlargement
   (b) Non-invasive tumor originating within the thymus
   (c) Waldenström macroglobulinemia
   (d) A and B
   (e) B and C
   (f) None of the above

40. **Indirect immunofluorescence on salt spit skin shows binding of the dermal (floor) side in all of the following conditions EXCEPT:**

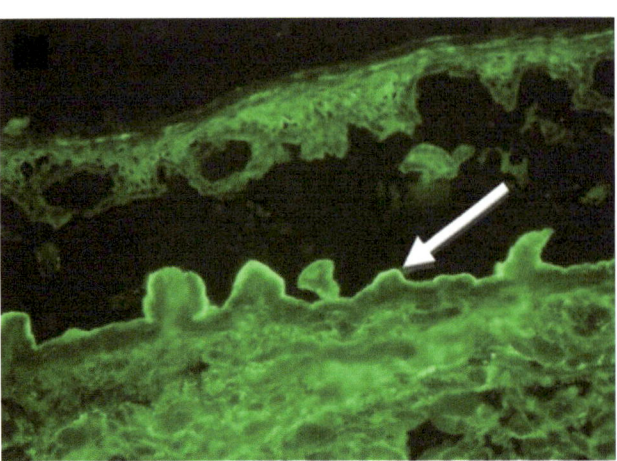

   (a) Bullous pemphigoid
   (b) Bullous lupus erythematosus
   (c) Anti-epiligrin cicatricial pemphigoid
   (d) Porphyria cutanea tarda

41. **Drug-induced subacute lupus erythematosus (SCLE) is most likely to be caused by the following:**
   (a) Hydralazine
   (b) Procainamide
   (c) Hydrochlorothiazide
   (d) Isoniazid

42. **A patient with the following cutaneous presentation but no systemic findings will have what approximate chance of progressing to systemic lupus erythematosus (SLE) over time?**

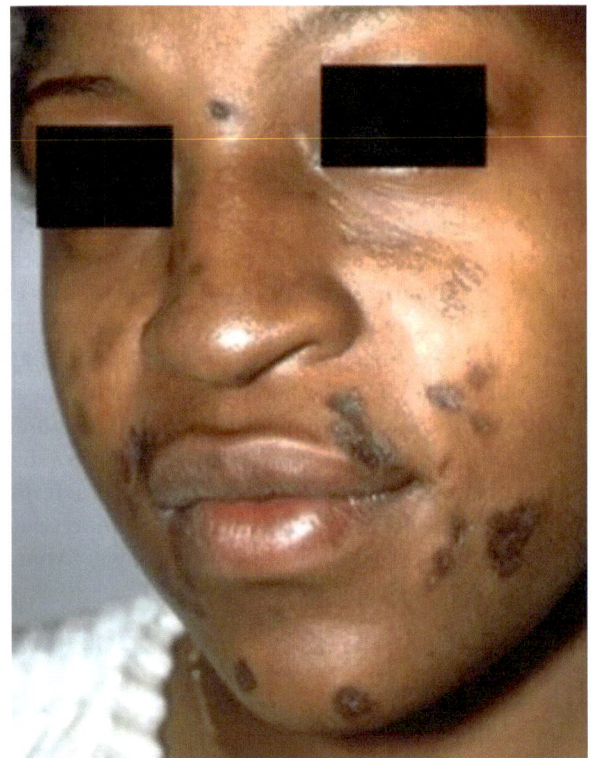

   (a) 5–15%
   (b) 80–90%
   (c) 30–50%
   (d) 50–70%

43. **What is the most frequent cause of increased both morbidity and mortality in a patient with muscle weakness, rash to the upper eyelids and poikiloderma to the lateral thighs?**
   (a) Cystic lung disease
   (b) Renal failure
   (c) Heart failure
   (d) Interstitial lung disease

44. **Which statement about dermatomyositis is not accurate?**
    (a) Scalp erythema, burning and/or poikiloderma with possible nonscarring alopecia can be seen in dermatomyositis patients, especially in women
    (b) There is an increased risk of cancer present but not typically seen within the first 5 years of diagnosis
    (c) The most common types of cancer in dermatomyositis include breast, ovarian, lung, gastrointestinal, and heme
    (d) The skin biopsy findings in dermatomyositis are similar to those found in systemic lupus erythematosus including vacuolar changes of the basal layer, increased lymphocytic infiltrate, and increased mucin deposition in the dermis
    (e) Clinical risk factors for malignancy include older age at onset and severe skin manifestations

45. **Which of the following is NOT an accurate statement regarding the likely diagnosis of a patient with hyperkeratosis of the palmar hands (specifically fingertips), arthralgias, and myalgias with shortness of breath?**
    (a) The antibodies are directed against aminoacyl transfer RNA synthetase
    (b) There is concern for interstitial lung disease
    (c) Anti-Jo-1 is the most common autoantibody seen in this syndrome
    (d) Anti-centromere autoantibodies are the most specific for the above syndrome

46. **The established prognostic markers for dermatomyositis that portend a poor prognosis include the following except:**
    (a) Cardiac involvement
    (b) Pulmonary disease
    (c) Mechanic's hands
    (d) Renal disease

47. **A 19-year-old girl has noticed asymptomatic bumps on the tip of her tongue that have increased in number over the past 1 year. They are painless but getting worse in number and size. She has no medical history and does not have similar bumps anywhere else on her body. You are most concerned about which of the following?**

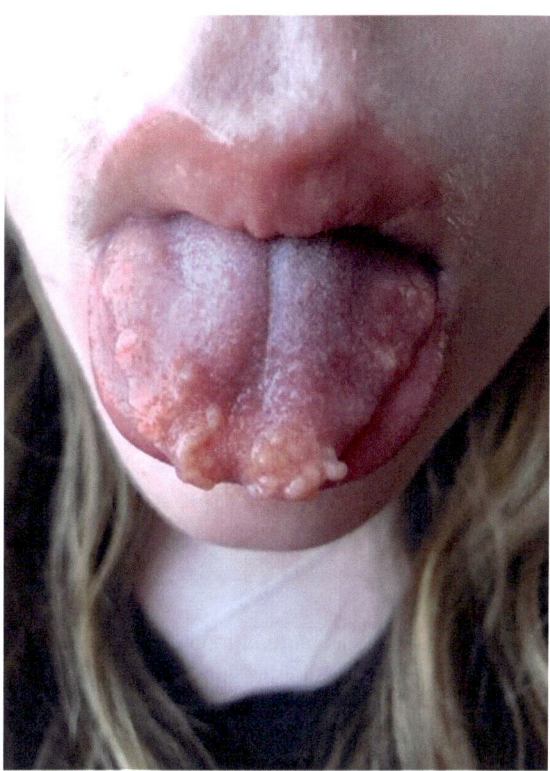

    (a) Underlying medullary thyroid carcinoma
    (b) Atrial myxomas causing heart failure
    (c) Underlying thyroid follicular carcinoma
    (d) Cushing syndrome

48. **Pemphigoid gestationis presents with pruritic urticarial papules on the trunk, especially the periumbilical region. This is unlike pruritic urticarial papules and plaques of pregnancy (PUPPP) in which the periumbilical area is typically spared.**
    (a) True
    (b) False

49. **The two dermatoses of pregnancy with increased risk to the baby are:**
    (a) Pemphigoid gestationis and PUPPP
    (b) Pemphigoid gestationis and cholestasis of pregnancy
    (c) Cholestasis of pregnancy and PUPPP
    (d) Prurigo of pregnancy and PUPPP
    (e) Prurigo of pregnancy and pemphigoid gestationis

50. **The antihistamine of choice for a pregnant patient is:**
    (a) Fexofenadine
    (b) Levocetirizine
    (c) Chlorpheniramine
    (d) Hydroxyzine

51. **A 19-year-old healthy female presents with painless discoloration to the abdomen for the past 6 months and she first noticed it after she started college. What is the most likely scenario?**

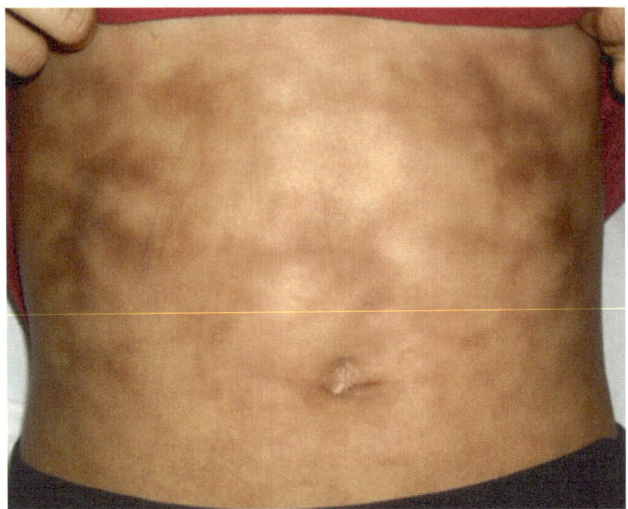

    (a) The patient has autoantibodies directed against phospholipid-binding proteins and has an increased risk of both thrombosis and pregnancy loss
    (b) The patient has an underlying non-inflammatory vasculopathy associated with headache, hypertension, and stroke
    (c) The patient is without any underlying issues and this is most likely due to the heat from her laptop chronically placed on her abdomen while lying in bed

52. **A 49-year-old male presents with asymptomatic erythema mainly to his neck that he noticed when he was outdoors playing golf about 1 year ago. He is not sure if it is worsening. What is the most likely diagnosis?**

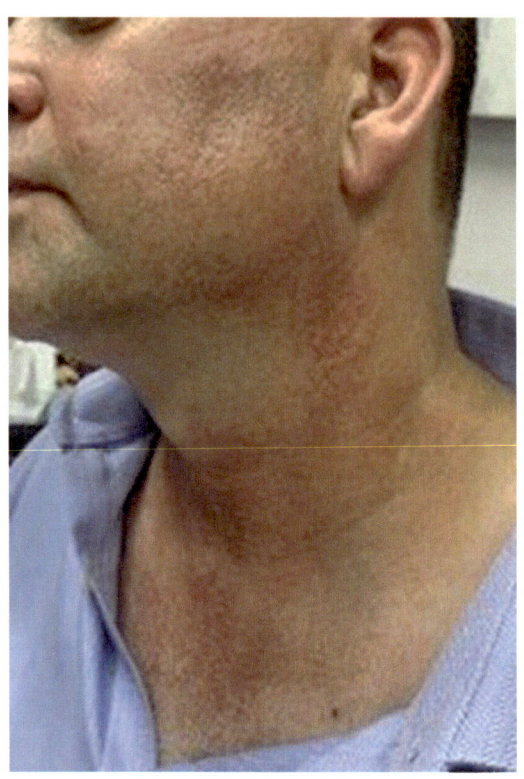

    (a) Contact dermatitis
    (b) Lupus erythematosus
    (c) Poikiloderma of Civatte
    (d) Riehl melanosis

53. **A 65-year-old female presents with a recurrent rash to her right cheek that occurs a few times per year over the past 5 years. She is not sure what might be causing it. The rash is asymptomatic and she denies any itching or pain when it appears. It goes away on its own after about 1 week. She is not any prescription medications but she is on a few over the counter medications on an as needed basis. Which of the following medications is the most likely culprit?**

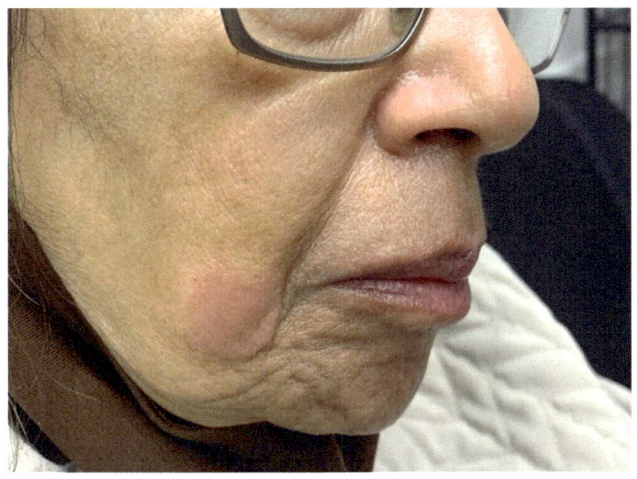

    (a) Naproxen
    (b) Famotidine
    (c) Cetirizine
    (d) Famotidine

54. **During a routine skin check, you see the lesion pictured here under the right breast. What is the most likely diagnosis?**

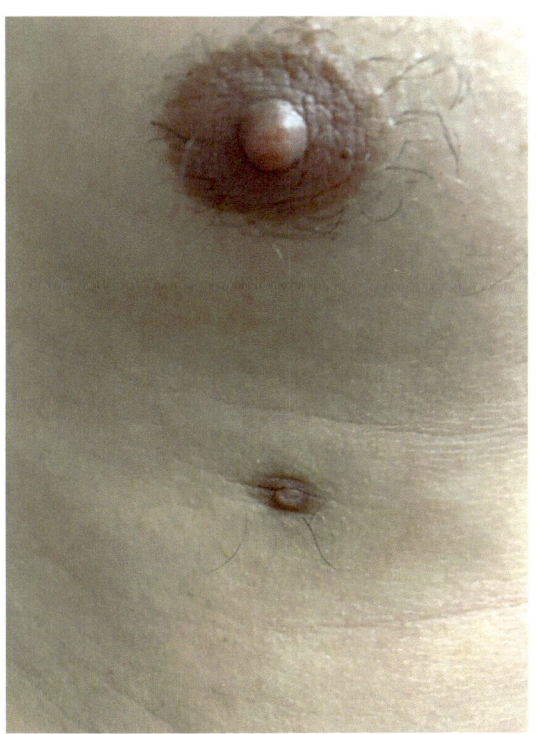

    (a) Acrochordon
    (b) Supernumerary nipple
    (c) Dermatofibroma
    (d) Melanocytic nevus
    (e) Neurofibroma

55. **A 48-year-old male presents with hypopigmentation bilaterally to his medial ventral wrists for the past 2 months. He states he has been having trouble with pain in his wrists and saw a hand surgeon 2–3 months ago and had an injection to the area but he cannot recall what medication was used. What is the most likely diagnosis of the discoloration?**

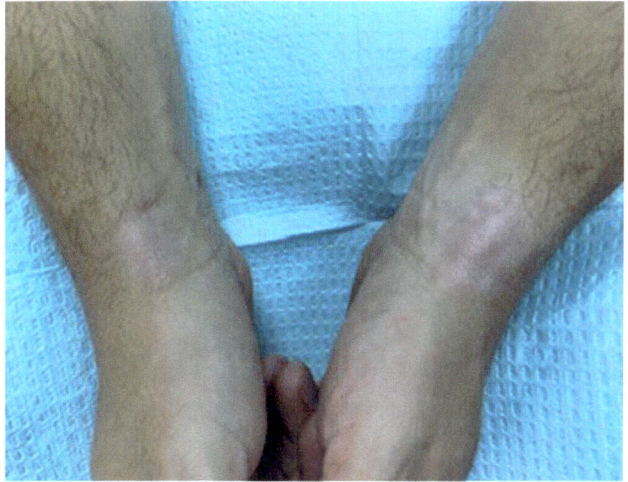

    (a) Hypopigmentation from a local corticosteroid injection
    (b) Vitiligo
    (c) Progressive macular hypomelanosis
    (d) Hypopigmented mycosis fungoides
    (e) Pressure-induced postinflammatory hypopigmentation

56. **How many gram(s) would be needed to apply a topical cream to the palmar surface of one hand?**
    (a) 5 g
    (b) 2 g
    (c) 1 g
    (d) 10 g

57. **A 65-year-old male presents for longstanding discoloration to his oral mucosa present for over 30 years. He also has discoloration to two fingers. He denies any similar findings in family members and no personal or family history of any type of cancer. He has had normal colonoscopies in the past and has been screened appropriately for his age. What is the next step?**

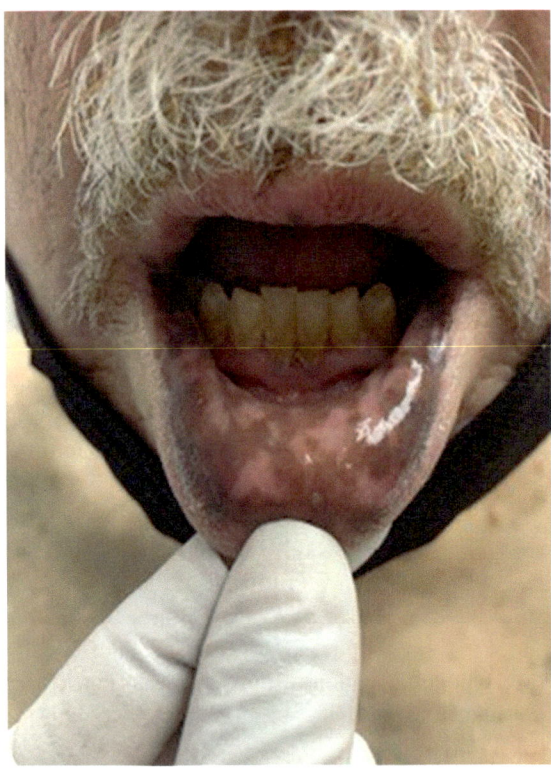

    (a) Advise the patient to increase the frequency of his colonoscopy to every 5 years instead of 10 as he will likely have an increased risk of colon cancer

    (b) Obtain an echocardiogram to rule out a possible atrial myxoma and potential heart failure

    (c) Obtain an electrocardiogram as the patient likely has hypertrophic cardiomyopathy

    (d) No further studies are needed as the patient likely has Laugier-Hunziker syndrome

58. **The best treatment for the condition pictured in the figure is:**

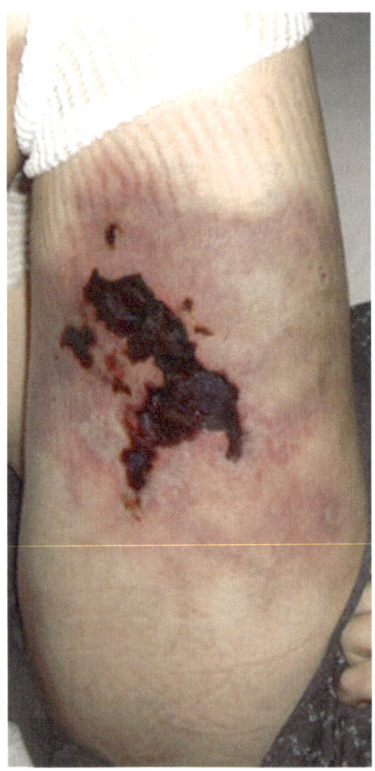

    (a) Sodium thiosulfate

    (b) Pentoxifylline

    (c) Saturated sodium potassium iodide (SSKI)

    (d) Hydroxychloroquine

59. **A 55-year-old female presents with a rash that she thinks started as an arthropod bite to her leg. She states it changed from a red small bump to a larger, painful ulcer. Which of the following statements is the most accurate regarding the patient's likely diagnosis?**

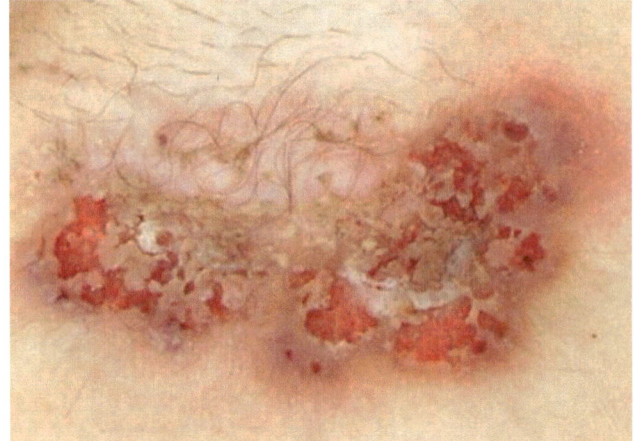

(a) The bullous variant is least likely associated with hematological diseases, such as myelogenous leukemia

(b) Direct immunofluorescence shows a linear band of IgG at the basement membrane

(c) It is associated with systemic diseases such as inflammatory bowel disease and hematological disorders

(d) Histopathology shows degeneration of the basal layer of the epidermis and a band-like lymphocytic infiltrate obscuring the dermoepidermal junction

60. **A 50-year-old male presents with acute erythema to his ear and states this has happened once before but it resolved on its own after 1 week. The area is painful and on further questioning, the patient also complains of migratory joint pain and intermittent irritation to his eyes. What is the concern if the above condition is untreated?**

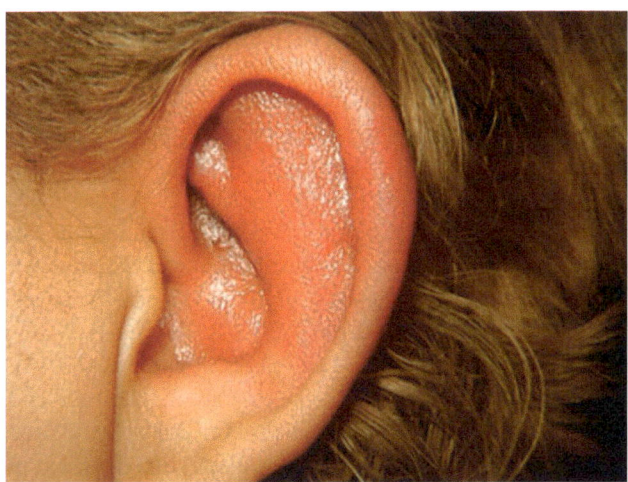

(a) Permanent deformity of the cartilage ("cauliflower ear" and saddle nose deformity)

(b) Posterior uveitis causing vision loss

(c) Superficial and deep thrombophlebitis

(d) Erosive sacroiliitis and pericarditis

Answer Key

For further information regarding the below answers, please see Chapter 3 of the corresponding *Dermatology: Illustrated Study Guide and Comprehensive Board Review, 3rd Edition* (2024).

1. **a**
2. **b**
3. **a**
4. **f**
5. **b**
6. **a**
7. **b**
8. **a**
9. **a**
10. **b**
11. **a**
12. **g**
13. **b**
14. **a**
15. **d**
16. **d**
17. **c**
18. **a**
19. **a**
20. **c**
21. **b**
22. **d**
23. **a**
24. **d**
25. **b**
26. **a**
27. **b**
28. **a**
29. **c**
30. **a**
31. **a**
32. **a**
33. **b**
34. **c**
35. **d**
36. **a**
37. **f**
38. **b**
39. **d**
40. **a**
41. **c**
42. **a**
43. **d**
44. **b**
45. **d**
46. **d**
47. **a**
48. **a**
49. **b**
50. **c**
51. **c**
52. **c**
53. **a**
54. **b**
55. **a**

56. **c**
57. **d**
58. **a**
59. **c**
60. **a**

Image Sources

3.1 Wu GY, Selsky N, Grant-Kels JM. Atlas of Dermatological Manifestations of Gastrointestinal Disease. New York: Springer; 2014. https://link.springer.com/chapter/10.1007/978-1-4614-6191-3_20

3.2 Hoekman, D.R., Roelofs, J.J.T.H., van Schuppen, J. et al. Case report of cheilitis granulomatosa and joint complaints as presentation of Crohn's disease. Clin J Gastroenterol 9, 73–78 (2016). https://doi.org/10.1007/s12328-016-0641-z. (Creative Commons Attribution 4.0 International License; http://creativecommons.org/licenses/by/4.0/)

3.4 Jain, S., Parikh, M.G. (2017). General Dermatology. In: Dermatology. Springer, Cham. https://doi.org/10.1007/978-3-319-47395-6_3

3.7 Walsh, R.K., Endicott, A.A. & Shinkai, K. Diagnosis and Treatment of Rosacea Fulminans: A Comprehensive Review. Am J Clin Dermatol 19, 79–86 (2018). https://doi.org/10.1007/s40257-017-0310-0

3.10 Phung, T.L., Wright, T.S., Pourciau, C.Y., Smoller, B.R. (2017). Interface Dermatoses. In: Pediatric Dermatopathology. Springer, Cham. https://doi.org/10.1007/978-3-319-44824-4_4

3.14 From Lie E, Sung S, Yang SH. Adult autoimmune enteropathy presenting initially with acquired Acrodermatitis Enteropathica: a case report. BMC Dermatol. 2017;17(7). https://doi.org/10.1186/s12895-017-0059-4 (Creative Commons Attribution 4.0 International License; http://creativecommons.org/licenses/by/4.0/)

3.26 Gonçalo, M. (2018). Phototoxic Dermatitis. In: John, S., Johansen, J., Rustemeyer, T., Elsner, P., Maibach, H. (eds) Kanerva's Occupational Dermatology. Springer, Cham. https://doi.org/10.1007/978-3-319-40221-5_15-2

3.34b Mutasim, D.F. (2008). Differential Diagnosis of Autoimmune Bullous Diseases in the Elderly. In: Norman, R.A. (eds) Diagnosis of Aging Skin Diseases. Springer, London. https://doi.org/10.1007/978-1-84628-678-0_10

3.38 Razera, F., Bonamigo, R.R. (2018). Paraneoplasias. In: Bonamigo, R., Dornelles, S. (eds) Dermatology in Public Health Environments. Springer, Cham. https://doi.org/10.1007/978-3-319-33919-1_46

3.40 Jain, S., Parikh, M.G. (2017). General Dermatology. In: Dermatology. Springer, Cham. https://doi.org/10.1007/978-3-319-47395-6_3

3.42 Jain, S., Parikh, M.G. (2017). General Dermatology. In: Dermatology. Springer, Cham. https://link.springer.com/chapter/10.1007/978-3-319-47395-6_3/figures/32

3.47 *Courtesy of* L. Greenberg MD

3.51 Phung, T.L., Wright, T.S., Pourciau, C.Y., Smoller, B.R. (2017). Interface Dermatoses. In: Pediatric Dermatopathology. Springer, Cham. https://doi.org/10.1007/978-3-319-44824-4_4

3.58 Phung, T.L., Wright, T.S., Pourciau, C.Y., Smoller, B.R. (2017). Deposition Disorders. In: Pediatric Dermatopathology. Springer, Cham. https://doi.org/10.1007/978-3-319-44824-4_16

3.59 Lipsker, D. (2013). Physical Examination in Dermatology: Primary Lesions. In: Clinical Examination and Differential Diagnosis of Skin Lesions. Springer, Paris. https://doi.org/10.1007/978-2-8178-0411-8_2

3.60 Krishnamurthy, A., Lee, D.H., Chan, A. (2013). Cutaneous Findings of Collagen Vascular Disease and Related Emergent Complications. In: Buka, B., Uliasz, A., Krishnamurthy, K. (eds) Buka's Emergencies in Dermatology. Springer, New York, NY. https://doi.org/10.1007/978-1-4614-5031-3_11

1. **What is the most likely diagnosis for the below painful eruption?**

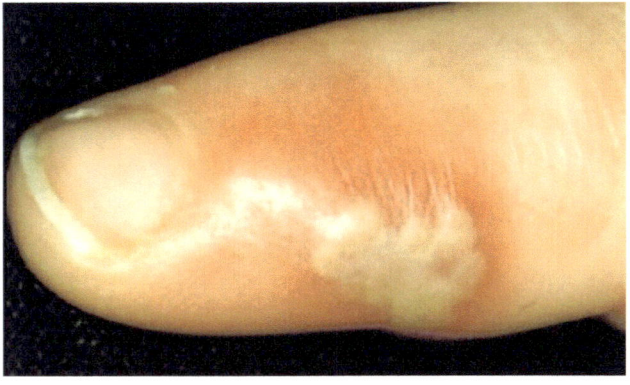

   (a) Herpetic whitlow
   (b) Dyshidrotic eczema
   (c) Contact dermatitis
   (d) Impetigo

2. **A herpes zoster rash involving the tip of the nose is important as this indicates which of the following:**
   (a) Facial nerve involvement with possible ocular involvement since the same nerve innervates the eye
   (b) Nasociliary nerve involvement with possible ocular involvement since the same nerve innervates the eye
   (c) Lacrimal nerve branch involvement with possible ocular involvement since the same nerve innervates the eye
   (d) Supratrochlear nerve involvement with possible ocular involvement since the same nerve innervates the eye

3. **Does a Tzanck smear differentiate between zoster and herpes simplex?**
   (a) Yes
   (b) No

4. **What is the most likely cause of this painful eruption seen below in this patient with a history of atopic dermatitis?**

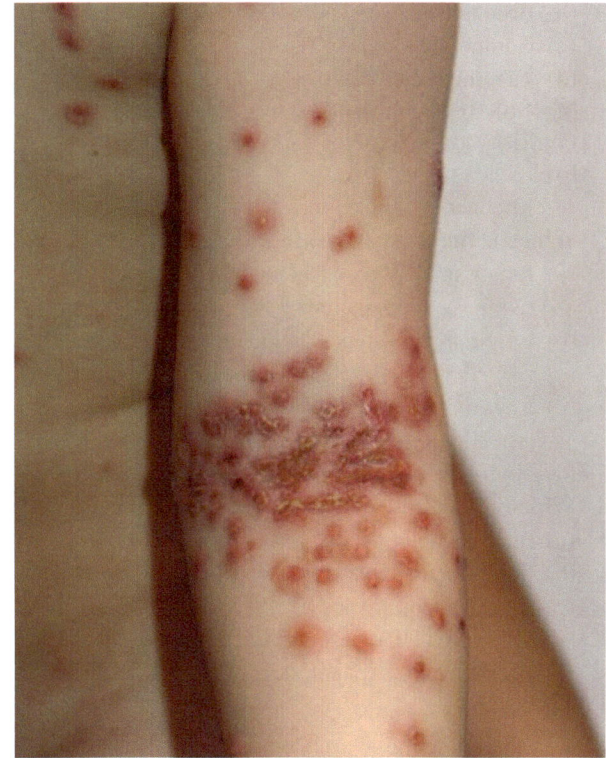

   (a) Eczema herpeticum
   (b) Dyshidrotic eczema
   (c) Contact dermatitis
   (d) Atopic dermatitis

5. **Human herpesvirus 8 (HHV8) has been associated with all of the following except:**
   (a) Primary effusion lymphoma
   (b) Castleman disease
   (c) Benign thymoma
   (d) Kaposi sarcoma

© The Author(s), under exclusive license to Springer Nature Switzerland AG 2024
S. Jain, *Dermatology High-Yield Self-Assessment*, https://doi.org/10.1007/978-3-031-73263-8_4

6. **A 25-year-old male who is sexually active presents with asymptomatic brownish-red papules on his penis for the past 6 months. He has no history of any lesions to the penis prior to this. What is the most likely diagnosis?**

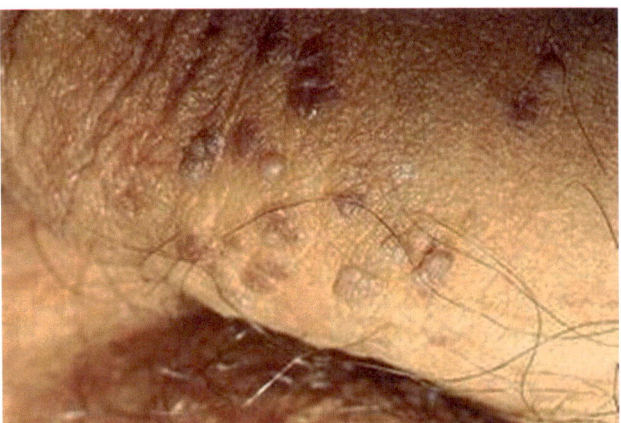

   (a) Bowenoid papulosis
   (b) Seborrheic keratosis
   (c) Flat warts
   (d) Lichen planus
   (e) Koebner phenomenon

7. **Which is the most accurate statement?**
   (a) Low-risk HPV types include 16 and 18, while high-risk HPV types include 6 and 11
   (b) Low-risk HPV types include 6 and 11, while high-risk HPV types include 16 and 18
   (c) Low-risk HPV types include 6 and 16, while high-risk HPV types include 11 and 18
   (d) High-risk HPV types include 6, 11, 16, and 18

8. **Which of the following is a live-attenuated vaccine?**
   (a) Intramuscular flu vaccine
   (b) Shingrix zoster vaccine
   (c) Zostavax zoster vaccine
   (d) Gardasil 9 HPV vaccine
   (e) Pneumovax 23 (pneumococcal vaccine polyvalent)

9. **What is the most likely diagnosis for the 5-year-old child with a painful rash shown in the figure? The rash is accompanied by painful defecation and blood-soaked stools.**

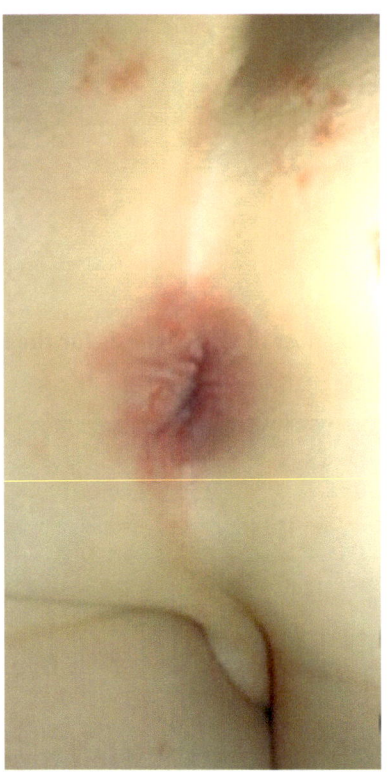

   (a) Erysipelas
   (b) Perianal streptococcal dermatitis
   (c) Erysipeloid
   (d) Pinworm infection

10. **A 15-year-old female presents with a "rash" on her feet as shown in the figure. She states she has been sweating more due to starting track at school and complains of malodor to her feet. On exam there are 1–2 mm punched-out areas. Which of the following is the best treatment for the condition?**

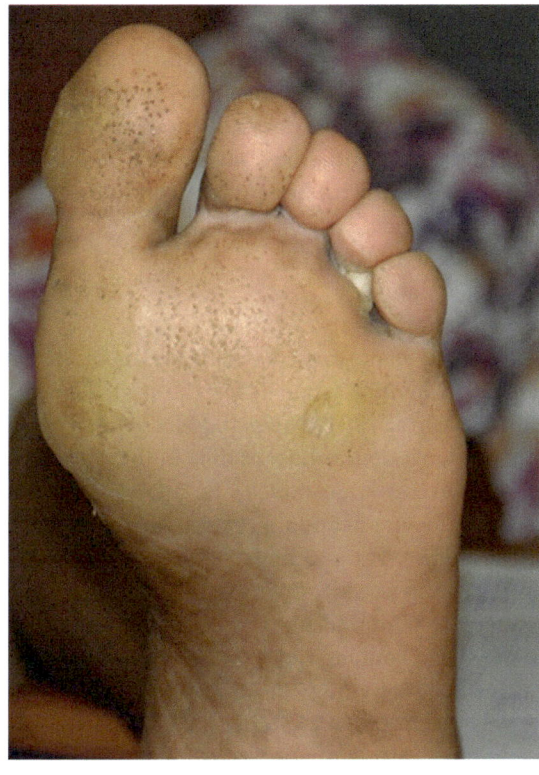

   (a) Topical antibiotic or benzoyl peroxide
   (b) Topical antifungal cream
   (c) Oral antifungal
   (d) Oral antibiotic

11. **What is the most likely cause of the frosted appearance to the axillae for the past 6 months?**

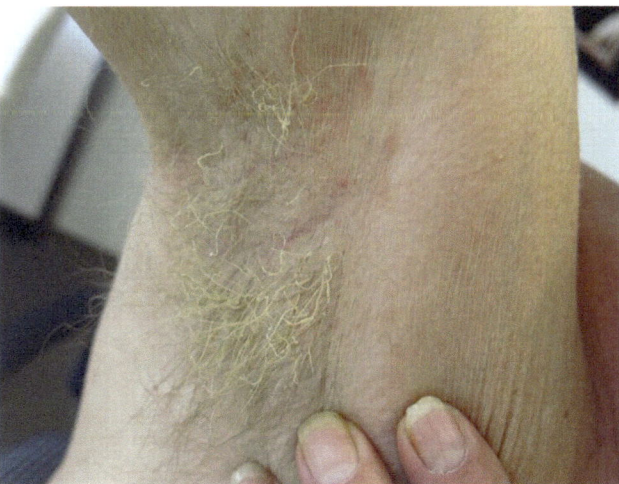

   (a) Corynebacterium minutissimum
   (b) Corynebacterium diphtheria
   (c) Erysipelothrix rhusiopathiae
   (d) Corynebacterium tenuis

12. **A 51-year-old male presents with a rash to his left dorsal hand for 2 weeks. The area became bright red and he has noticed that the affected area has expanded in the past 1 week. He has a moderate amount of alcohol regularly. His hobbies are cooking and fishing and he states before the rash started, he went fishing and his left hand was wounded by a fishbone. What is the best treatment for this rash?**

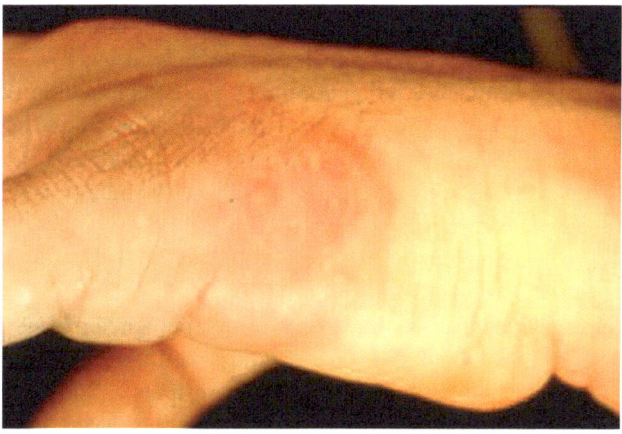

   (a) Cephalosporin
   (b) Combination of sulfamethoxazole and trimethoprim
   (c) Ciprofloxacin
   (d) Clindamycin
   (e) Doxycycline

13. **A 13-year-old female with no past medical history presents with a tender nodule to her left preauricular region for past 3 weeks. After further questioning, she states her family bought a new kitten about 5 weeks ago. During your review of systems, the patient was positive for fatigue and intermittent achiness. What is the most accurate statement regarding the diagnosis?**

   (a) An oral antibiotic, specifically azithromycin, is needed in this case as it typically does not self-resolve in healthy or immunosuppressed patients
   (b) It may happen with contact through a bite or scratch from a cat infected by fleas with Bartonella bacilliformis
   (c) Cat scratch disease typically happens within 24 h from time of the infected scratch
   (d) No treatment in this patient's case is necessary as this typically resolves on its own in healthy patients

14. **A 55-year-old man presented to the emergency department with high fever, chills, and excruciating pain in his left fifth finger. The only thing he remembers earlier that day is that he unexpectedly punctured his fifth left finger on the fin of a Japanese sea perch when he selected fish at the market earlier that morning. By evening time, he felt itching to his finger and it started to swell. A few hours later, he had a fever and chills and severe pain to the finger. What is the most likely culprit?**
    (a) *Vibrio vulnificus*
    (b) *Pseudomonas aeruginosa*
    (c) *Bartonella bacilliformis*
    (d) Parapoxvirus (Orfviridae)

15. **A 12-year-old boy scout returned from a summer camping trip 1 week ago presents with high fever, lethargy, headache, and abdominal pain. Petechial lesions are seen on his palms and feet but his mother states the lesions initially started on his wrists and ankles. What is the most appropriate treatment for this diagnosis?**
    (a) Doxycycline
    (b) Rifampicin
    (c) Ciprofloxacin
    (d) Combination of trimethoprim and sulfamethoxazole

16. **The mother of the child in question 15 is pregnant and also presents with similar symptoms as her son. She has an allergy to tetracyclines. What is the best treatment option for her?**
    (a) Rifampicin
    (b) Azithromycin
    (c) Doxycycline
    (d) Chloramphenicol

17. **A false positive rapid plasma reagin (RPR) may be seen in all of the following cases except:**
    (a) Rickettsial infection
    (b) Pregnancy
    (c) Tuberculosis
    (d) Systemic lupus erythematosus (SLE)
    (e) Diabetes

18. **Which of the following scenarios is the least accurate regarding testing for syphilis?**
    (a) If screening rapid plasma reagin (RPR) is positive, confirmation should be checked with fluorescent treponemal antibody absorption test (FTA-ABS)
    (b) Reactivity to a treponemal test (FTA-ABS) implies infection but does not determine whether the infection is recent or remote, and it also will stay positive even after syphilis has been successfully treated
    (c) Unlike RPR and venereal disease research laboratory (VDRL), the confirmatory test FTA-ABS never has false positives
    (d) Negative RPR but positive FTA-ABS is consistent with a prior infection of syphilis
    (e) Chronic false positive VDRL lasting great than 6 months can be seen in patients with systemic lupus erythematosus

19. **A 30-year-old female presents with fever and multiple tender erythematous ulcerated nodules over the body but concentrated over legs and arms for the past 3 weeks. Of note, the patient states she was recently diagnosed with leprosy and for the past 3 months has been on multidrug therapy (dapsone, rifampicin, clofazimine along oral prednisone) and she was doing well until recently. Prednisone has not been able to be tapered down as she gets new crops of lesions when tried in the past. Biopsy shows necrotizing vasculitis of the vessels of the deep dermis and subcutis. What is the best medication to add to this regimen to help with her current condition?**
    (a) Thalidomide
    (b) Pentoxifylline
    (c) Azathioprine
    (d) Methotrexate

20. **40-year-old male presents with an enlarged tender nodule to his left forearm for the past 4 weeks. He thinks the area is enlarging and has noticed two similar smaller lesions adjacent to it in the past 2 weeks. When further questioned, he states he recently returned from vacation in Costa Rica where he was scuba diving. He accidentally hit a sea urchin with his left forearm while trying to take a picture. He had immediate pain and noticed a few sea urchin spines to the site of contact, but he was seen by a local medical facility soon after. The spines were removed, and he was given tetanus vaccination and 1 week of oral cephalexin. A few weeks later he started noticing an enlarging nodule at site of contact with the sea urchin and a few new lesions as pictured below. What is most likely the culprit?**

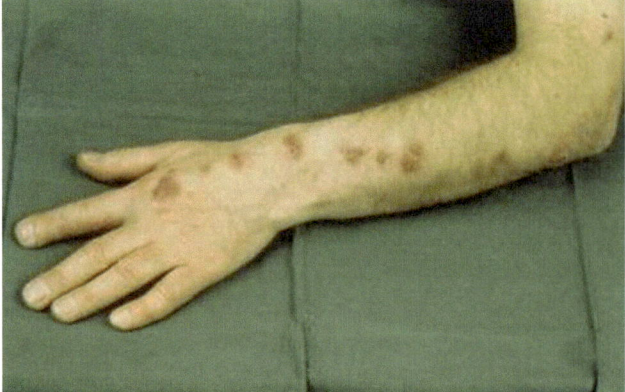

    (a) *Mycobacterium marinum*
    (b) *Ecthyma gangrenosum*
    (c) *Mycobacterium leprae*
    (d) *Mycobacterium kansasii*

21. **A patient presents with smooth painless nodules after going on vacation in Mexico and swimming in the ocean where he saw dolphins and whales. What is a characteristic feature you might see on histology in such a patient?**
    (a) Round or lemon-shaped cells attached to one another with narrow connections ("chain of coins" or "brass knuckles")
    (b) Dark-colored, thick-walled muriform bodies (medlar bodies or "copper pennies")
    (c) Thick, double-contoured wall with broad-based budding
    (d) Round central cell with multiple buds attached by narrow necks ("mariner's wheel")

22. **A healthy 55-year-old male with no past medical history and lives in Chicago, Illinois presents with a verrucous skin-colored plaque on his dorsal foot for the past 3 months that is slowly enlarging. The area is asymptomatic and he feels well. What is the most likely diagnosis?**

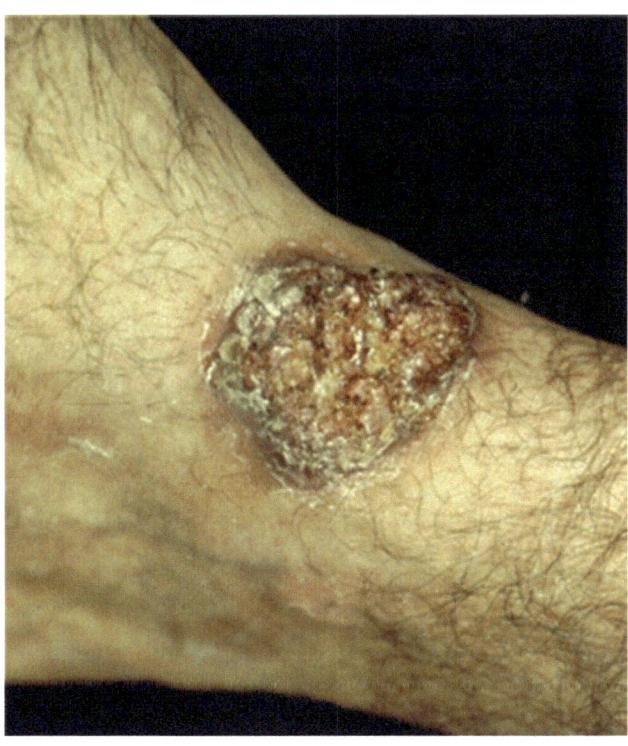

    (a) Lobomycosis
    (b) Blastomycosis
    (c) Paracoccidioidomycosis
    (d) Cryptococcosis

23. **What is the least accurate statement about *Mycobacterium leprae*?**
    (a) *M. leprae* differs from other mycobacteria in that this species cannot be cultured in vitro (does not grow in artificial media)
    (b) *M. leprae* can be cultivated in artificial media but needs a higher temperature than other mycobacteria species and requires minimum of 5 months to grow
    (c) The nine-banded armadillo is the only known natural non-human vertebrate host of *M. leprae*
    (d) A susceptible individual, once infected, often exhibits an incubation period of typically 3–7 years until symptoms are observed
    (e) Transmission occurs through continuous and close contact of susceptible people with untreated infected people

24. **A 45-year-old female who moved here from Costa Rica 3 years ago presents with a 2-year history of an erythematous nontender nodule to her L lower cheek that is not growing in size. She states she has been very busy with the move and you are the first doctor she has seen in the past 3 years. What is next step to determine the diagnosis?**

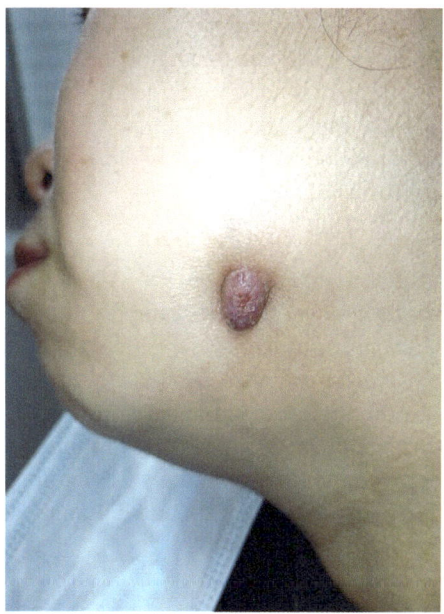

    (a) Empiric treatment with shave removal and electrodessication as this is a common, acquired, benign vascular tumor that typically presents as a red, friable solitary papule
    (b) Check her teeth as this is likely a purulent by-product of dental pulp necrosis spread along the path of least resistance from the root apex to the skin of the face
    (c) Perform a skin biopsy and send for tissue culture as this is likely a mycobacterial infection
    (d) Give her an antibiotic to decrease inflammation as she likely she has a ruptured epidermal inclusion cyst

25. **65-year-old man presents with a rash on his body including red nodules on his arms for the past 1 year. He initially noticed painless red bumps on his upper arms that progressed to his abdomen and chest. He has seen other physicians for this in the past and was told the 3 biopsies performed were all inconclusive. Around the same time as the rash began, he noticed a progressive ulcer on his lower leg that he is still being treated for by the wound clinic. The wound is much smaller now and he is only taking prednisone 20 mg daily for this. He has not traveled outside the United States in the past 8 years. Patient has also noticed decreased sensation to hot and cold temperatures with his hands in the past year or so. What is the most likely etiology of his rash and above symptoms?**

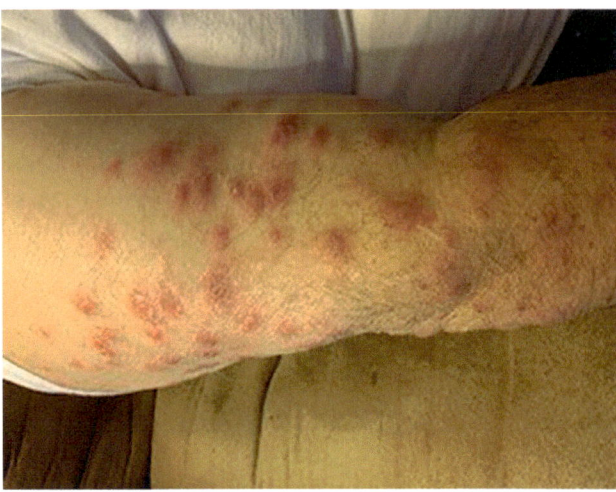

   (a) *Mycobacterium marinum*
   (b) *Mycobacterium chelonae* complex
   (c) *Mycobacterium leprae*
   (d) *Mycobacterium kansasii*

26. **What is the most likely diagnosis in this 14-year-old healthy female with a pruritic, annular scaly erythematous patch approximately 2.5 cm in diameter, growing centrifugally on the medial angle of the left eyelid for the past 1 month?**

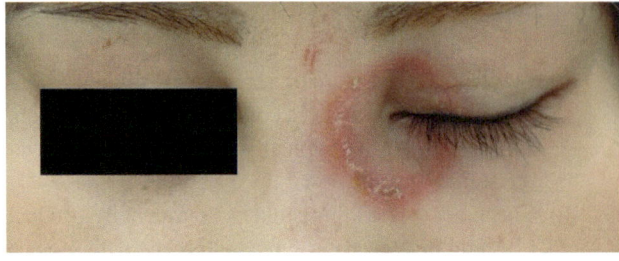

   (a) Tinea faciei
   (b) Atopic dermatitis
   (c) Allergic contact dermatitis
   (d) Nummular dermatitis

27. **A 7-year-old female presents with an itchy rash mainly to her face and arms for the past 1 month. On examination, she has multiple skin-colored small monomorphic bumps mainly to her face. She also has enlarged posterior cervical lymph nodes and focal scaling with associated hair loss to her scalp. On further questioning, the patient's mother states that she has had a scaly area on her scalp for quite some time. What is the most likely reason for her rash?**

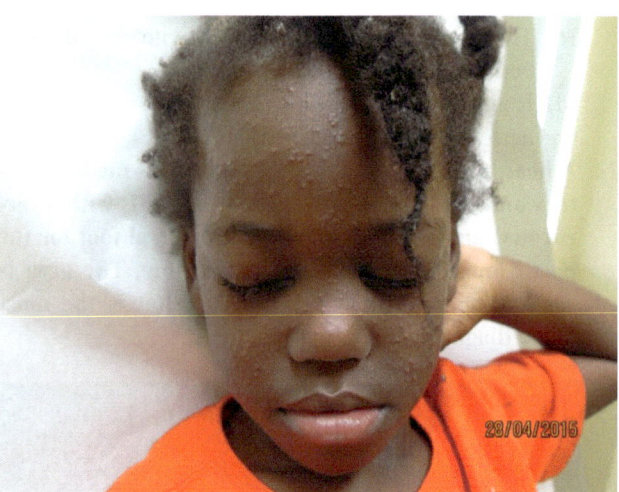

   (a) Atopic dermatitis from uncontrolled seborrheic dermatitis
   (b) Autoeczematization or id reaction from psoriasis to the scalp
   (c) Autoeczematization or id reaction from pre-existing tinea capitis
   (d) Viral eruption and unrelated but concomitant tinea capitis

28. **What is the first-line treatment for a pregnant female patient with scabies?**
   (a) Topical crotamiton
   (b) Topical permethrin
   (c) Oral ivermectin
   (d) Topical ivermectin

29. **What is most common dermatophyte causing distal subungual onychomycosis?**
   (a) *Trichophyton rubrum*
   (b) *Trichophyton mentagrophytes*
   (c) *Trichophyton tonsurans*
   (d) *Trichophyton concentricum*

30. **A 20-year-old sexually active female presented with a worsening nonpruritic rash on her palms and soles for 1 month duration. She denies any fever, pain, pruritus, dysuria, vaginal discharge or previous vaginal sores. On further investigation, she admits to being treated in the emergency department for gonorrhea last year. What is the best treatment for this diagnosis?**

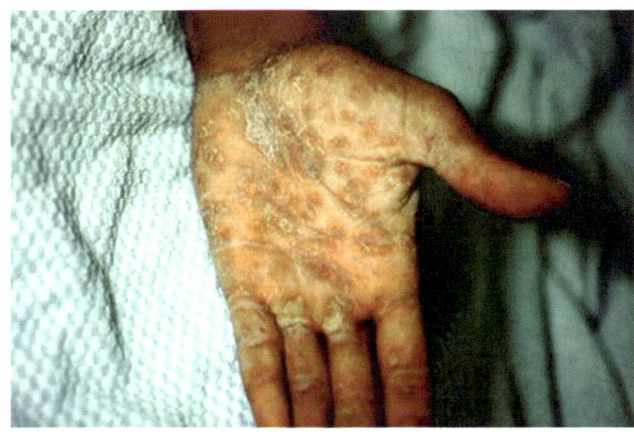

(a) Clindamycin 300 mg twice daily and rifampicin 300 mg daily for 6 weeks
(b) A single injection of long-acting benzathine penicillin G
(c) Doxycycline 100 mg twice daily for 3 weeks
(d) Cephalexin 2000 mg as a one-time dose

31. **A 30-year-old female with a history of recent travel history to Belize and Guatemala presented with a red area with associated swelling and pruritus near her shoulder for 2 weeks after returning to the USA. During her trip, the patient, accompanied by her family, visited many forests, lakes, rivers, and sulfur hot springs. While in those countries, she reported multiple mosquito bites despite taking protective measures. Which infectious etiology will be in your differential due to her travel history and her presentation?**

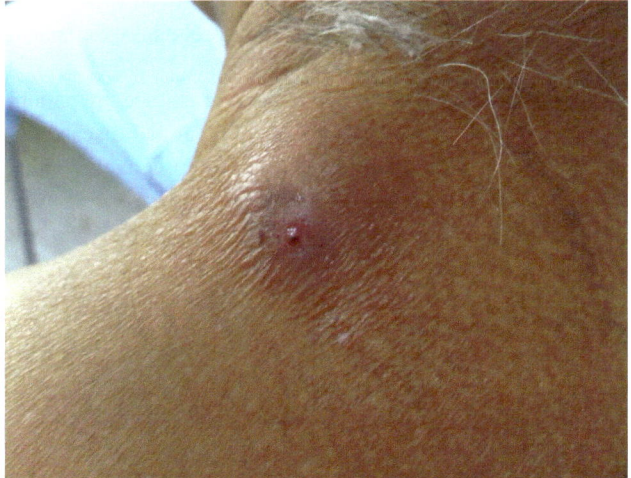

(a) *Strongyloides stercoralis*
(b) *Onchocerca volvulus*
(c) *Mycobacterium abscessus*
(d) *Dermatobia hominis*
(e) *Entamoeba histolytica*

32. **An 18-year-old male presented with an intensely pruritic eruption on the buttocks, thighs and trunk. On further questioning his mother states they were on vacation and went snorkeling and even went scuba diving for the first time. The itching started 1 day after snorkeling and the pruritus is keeping him up at night. What is the most likely cause of the eruption?**
(a) Due to brushing against jellyfish tentacles
(b) Due to free-swimming infectious cercariae of avian schistosomes
(c) Due to exposure to the larval form of thimble jellyfish (*Linuche unguiculata*) and sea anemone (*Edwardsiella lineata*) that become entrapped underneath swimwear

33. **Which deep fungal infection is associated with pigeon droppings and shows a zone of clearance or "halo" around the cells when stained with India ink under the microscope?**
(a) Blastomycosis
(b) Histoplasmosis
(c) Cryptococcosis
(d) Coccidioidomycosis

34. **A 90-year-old man who recently moved here from Turkey and with chronic venous insufficiency and benign prostatic hyperplasia presents with multiple erythematous plaques and patches to lower legs over the past 2 years. They are painless and he states he started with one area but has now spread. What will most likely be seen on histopathology?**

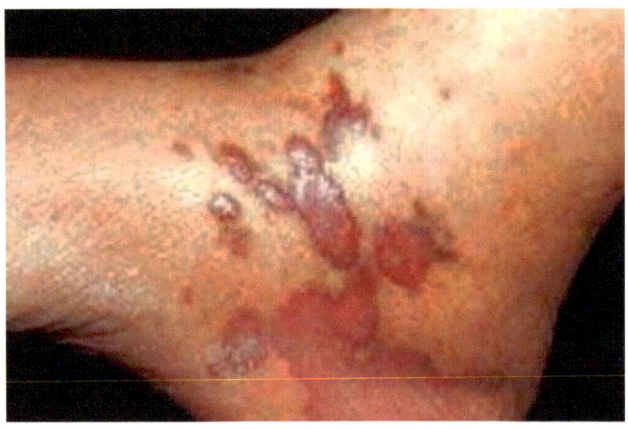

(a) Increased spindle-shaped cells with vascular slits and vascular structures with predominance of endothelial cells, extravasated erythrocytes and hemosiderin-laden macrophages

(b) Marked proliferation of small-caliber vessels, lymphoid hyperplasia and the presence of many eosinophils in the background

(c) Capillaritis in the dermis with concomitant venous hypertension leading to endothelial cell dysfunction and extravasation of red blood cells

(d) Extravasation of red blood cells only

35. **Which two statements are the most accurate regarding bed bugs?**

(a) They are invisible to the naked eye

(b) They hide in dark, warm places like mattresses, box springs, carpet, behind headboards, and cracks in the wall

(c) Indirect visible signs can prove helpful in their detection and include fecal specks and blood stains

(d) They forage during the day and night and the peak time to find them is around 7 pm

(e) The areas most affected by bed bug bites include the chest, back and proximal extremities

(f) It is characteristic to see three small round bite marks located a few centimeters apart in a linear fashion ("breakfast, lunch, and dinner") in non-exposed areas such as the chest and groin

36. **A 61-year-old man presented with a pruritic, erythematous scaly rash of 2 weeks duration involving the scrotum and both inguinal creases. Under examination with ultraviolet A light from a Wood's lamp, the rash exhibited a coral-red fluorescence. This color is due to:**

(a) Overproduction of coproporphyrin III by *Corynebacterium minutissimum*

(b) Overproduction of coproporphyrin III by *Corynebacterium tenuis*

(c) Overproduction of pteridine by *Microsporum audouinii*

(d) Overproduction of pyoverdine by *Pseudomonas aeruginosa*

37. **A 22-year-old male presented with a 9-month history of white clumps on the hair shafts of his axillae. Yellow-green fluorescence was seen on Wood's lamp examination. Which one of the following statements is not accurate regarding the diagnosis?**

(a) Malodor from the infection is related to bacterial metabolism of testosterone

(b) The infection is related to *Corynebacterium* spp. (*C. tenuis*) that colonize the hair shaft of the axilla

(c) The infection is related to a fungus (*Trichosporon* spp.) that colonizes the hair shaft of the axilla

(d) Dermoscopy reveals waxy yellowish-white or brown nodules and concretions adherent to the hair

(e) Wood's lamp exam reveals weak yellowish fluorescence

(f) Complete resolution by general hygiene measures such as shaving off all axillary hairs and maintaining the area dry along with topical treatment such topical benzoyl peroxide, erythromycin or clindamycin can expedite clearance and prevent recurrence

38. **Which of the following is the most accurate statement regarding treatment for Lyme disease when early, localized disease?**

(a) Doxycycline is the treatment of choice in patients older than 8 years with early localized disease but amoxicillin should be used for pregnant women and children under 8 years

(b) Amoxicillin is the treatment of choice in patient older than 8 years with early localized disease but doxycycline should be used for pregnant women and children under 8 years

(c) Doxycycline is the treatment of choice for all patients

(d) Ceftriaxone is the treatment for all adults, including pregnant women

39. **What is the mainstay treatment for mucocutaneous leishmaniasis?**
    (a) Sodium thiosulfate
    (b) Sodium stibogluconate
    (c) Diethylcarbamazine
    (d) Ivermectin

40. **What is the concern of starting a patient with onchocerciasis on oral diethylcarbamazine?**
    (a) Lucio reaction
    (b) Mazzotti reaction
    (c) Jarisch–Herxheimer reaction
    (d) Reversal reaction

41. **The following finding on Wood's lamp examination in a young patient complaining of a foul-smelling rash on his feet would support which causative agent?**

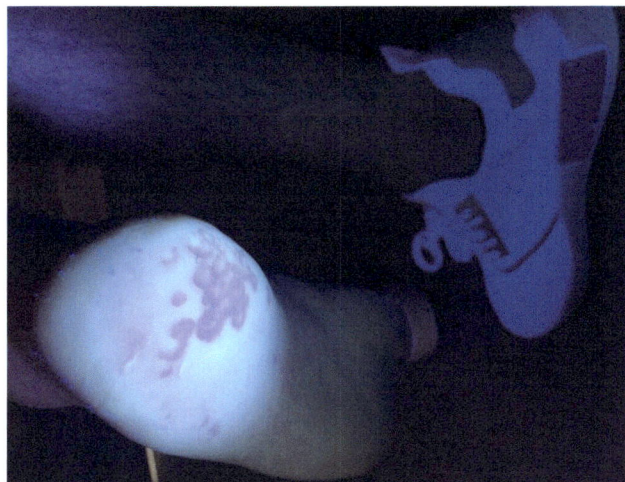

    (a) *Corynebacterial* infection
    (b) *Staphylococcal* infection
    (c) *Streptococcal* infection
    (d) *E. coli* infection

Answer Key

For further information regarding the below answers, please see Chapter 4 of the corresponding *Dermatology: Illustrated Study Guide and Comprehensive Board Review, 3rd Edition* (2024).

1. **a**
2. **b**
3. **b**
4. **a**
5. **c**
6. **a**
7. **b**
8. **c**
9. **b**
10. **a**
11. **d**
12. **a**
13. **d**
14. **a**
15. **a**
16. **d**
17. **e**
18. **c**
19. **a**
20. **a**
21. **a**
22. **b**
23. **b**
24. **b**
25. **c**
26. **a**
27. **c**
28. **b**
29. **a**
30. **b**
31. **d**
32. **c**
33. **c**
34. **a**
35. **b and c**
36. **a**
37. **c**
38. **a**
39. **b**
40. **b**
41. **a**

Image Sources

4.1 Nikkels, A.F., Pièrard, G.E. Treatment of Mucocutaneous Presentations of Herpes Simplex Virus Infections. Am J Clin Dermatol 3, 475–487 (2002). https://doi.org/10.2165/00128071-200203070-00004

4.4 Damour A, Garcia M, Seneschal J, Lévêque N, Bodet C. Eczema Herpeticum: Clinical and Pathophysiological Aspects. Clin Rev Allergy Immunol. 2020 Aug;59(1):1–18. https://doi.org/10.1007/s12016-019-08768-3. PMID: 31836943.

4.6 Gloster HM, Gebauer LE, Mistur RL. Viral Infections. In: Absolute Dermatology Review. Cham, Switzerland: Springer; 2016. pp 221–233. https://doi.org/10.1007/978-3-319-03218-4_53

4.9 Jongen J, Eberstein A, Peleikis HG, Kahlke V, Herbst RA. Perianal streptococcal dermatitis: an important differential diagnosis in pediatric patients. Dis Colon Rectum. 2008 May;51(5):584–7. https://doi.org/10.1007/s10350-008-9237-0. Epub 2008 Mar 7. PMID: 18324440.

4.10 Naafs, B., Dassoni, F., Morrone, A. (2020). Bacterial Dermatoses. In: Morrone, A., Hay, R., Naafs, B. (eds) Skin Disorders in Migrants. Springer, Cham. https://doi.org/10.1007/978-3-030-37476-1_4

4.11 Wollina, U. (2020). Yellowish Axillary Hair. In: Lotti, T., Tirant, M., Parsad, D. (eds) Clinical Cases in Pigmentary Disorders. Clinical Cases in Dermatology. Springer, Cham. https://doi.org/10.1007/978-3-030-50823-4_44

4.12 Bonamonte, D., Filoni, A., Vestita, M., Angelini, G. (2016). Cutaneous Infections from Aquatic Environments. In: Bonamonte, D., Angelini, G. (eds) Aquatic Dermatology. Springer, Cham. https://doi.org/10.1007/978-3-319-40615-2_11

4.20 Petrini, B. Mycobacterium marinum: ubiquitous agent of waterborne granulomatous skin infections. Eur J Clin Microbiol Infect Dis 25, 609–613 (2006). https://doi.org/10.1007/s10096-006-0201-4

4.22 Gloster, H.M., Gebauer, L.E., Mistur, R.L. (2016). Fungal Infections. In: Absolute Dermatology Review. Springer, Cham. https://doi.org/10.1007/978-3-319-03218-4_54

4.24 Fang, R., Wang, L., Yang, R., Li, S., Li, Y. (2022). A Female in Middle Age with Red Nodule. In: Lotti, T.M., Jafferany, M., Gao, XH., Abdelmaksoud, A. (eds) Clinical Cases in Facial Erythema. Clinical Cases in Dermatology. Springer, Cham. https://doi.org/10.1007/978-3-031-05996-4_5

4.26 Shimoyama, H., Yo, A., Makimura, K. et al. A Case of Tinea faciei Due to Nannizzia gypsea: Inflammatory Eruption on the Medial Angle of the Eyelid. Mycopathologia 185, 699–703 (2020). https://doi.org/10.1007/s11046-020-00474-5

4.30 Kinser, K., Dominguez, A.R. (2014). Syphilis. In: Jackson-Richards, D., Pandya, A. (eds) Dermatology Atlas for Skin of Color. Springer, Berlin, Heidelberg. https://doi.org/10.1007/978-3-642-54446-0_36

4.31 Wikipedia. https://en.wikipedia.org/wiki/Myiasis#/media/File:Miasis_human.jpg (public domain: https://creativecommons.org/publicdomain/zero/1.0/deed.en)

4.34 Gloster, H.M., Gebauer, L.E., Mistur, R.L. Kaposi's Sarcoma. In: Absolute Dermatology Review. Springer Cham: Springer; 2016. pp. 379. https://doi.org/10.1007/978-3-319-03218-4_87

Benign and Malignant Tumors

1. A 12-year-old healthy male presents with a 2-year history of multiple skin-colored papules to the central face that are both smooth and firm. The lesions are asymptomatic. He has no family history of cancer and the patient's mother states no one in the family has similar lesions. Which of the following is the most likely mutation in this case?

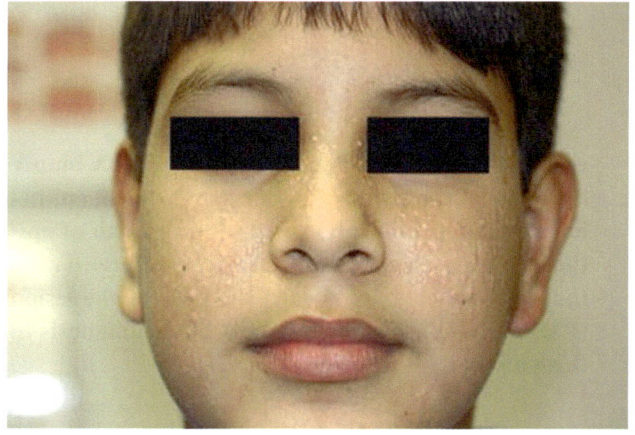

  (a) CYLD gene mutation
  (b) PTEN gene mutation
  (c) RET gene mutation
  (d) c-KIT mutation

2. A 22-year-old male presents with a 1-cm pink nodule to the right postauricular region. Histology shows solid nests of basaloid cells undergoing abrupt trichilemmal-type keratinization, ghost cells, calcification, and foreign body reaction. On further questioning, the patient mentions he has had similar lesions and he thinks this is the eighth one he has had so far. Which of the following conditions would not be part of your differential given his history?

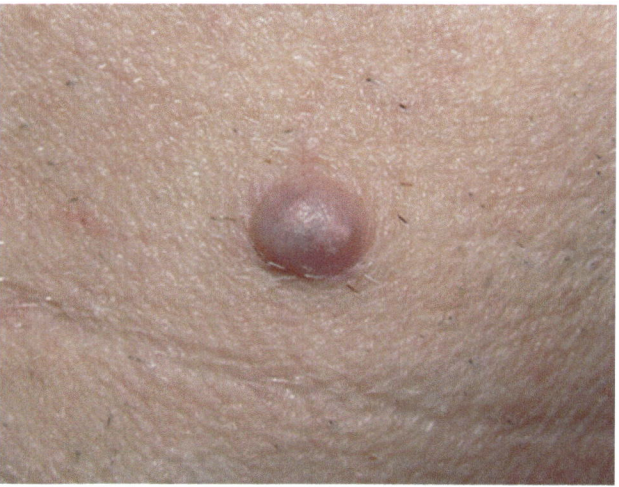

  (a) Rubinstein-Taybi syndrome
  (b) Gardner syndrome
  (c) Myotonic dystrophy
  (d) Cowden syndrome

© The Author(s), under exclusive license to Springer Nature Switzerland AG 2024
S. Jain, *Dermatology High-Yield Self-Assessment*, https://doi.org/10.1007/978-3-031-73263-8_5

3. **A 24-year-old female presents with small bumps on the tip of her tongue for the past year that have increased in number. They are asymptomatic but she complains of accidentally biting them often at rest. Her past medical history includes a new diagnosis of hypertension and palpitations. You perform a 24-h urine test to check her catecholamine level which is positive. What other lab test might be elevated in this patient?**

(a) Parathyroid hormone
(b) Thyroid stimulating hormone
(c) Calcitonin
(d) Phosphorus

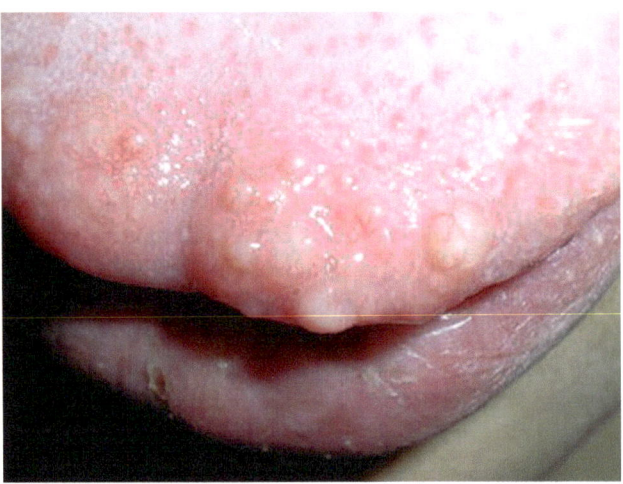

4. **A 15-year-old male presents with his mother with multiple skin-colored papules to his face, especially along the chin and jawline, that have increased in number over the past 2 years. The lesions are asymptomatic and have been treated as acne in the past without any improvement. The patient's mother states her husband had similar lesions and was diagnosed with cancer of the thyroid. A biopsy from one of the lesions shows a symmetrical epithelial nodular proliferation with downgrowth of epithelial cells with increasing clear cell differentiation that is more obvious toward the base of the lesion (PAS positive). What is the most likely diagnosis in this patient?**

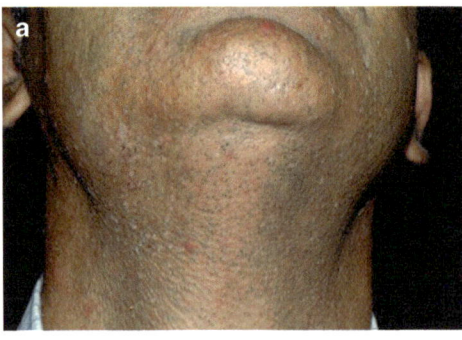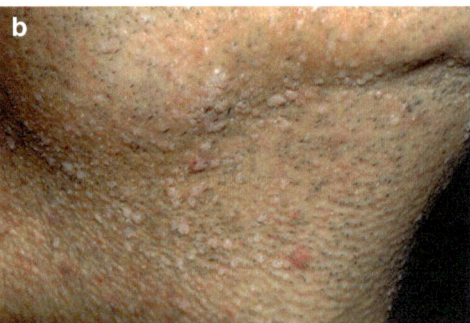

(a) Gardner syndrome
(b) Birt-Hogg-Dubé syndrome
(c) Tuberous sclerosis
(d) Cowden syndrome

5. **A 65-year-old man presents to clinic for a second opinion. He has noticed more bumps on his face in the past 3 years. They are asymptomatic. He has a biopsy report that is consistent with a fibrofolliculoma. On further questioning, he states his father was diagnosed with lung cysts and had recurrent spontaneous pneumothorax. What would you be concerned about with this patient?**
   (a) An underlying gastric adenocarcinoma
   (b) Lymphangioleiomyomatosis
   (c) Underlying renal cancer
   (d) Breast cancer

6. **Which of the following is the most common neoplasm seen within a nevus sebaceous from the options listed below?**
   (a) Trichoblastoma
   (b) Basal cell carcinoma
   (c) Trichofolliculoma
   (d) Hidradenoma papilliferum

7. **A 20-year-old healthy male with no past medical history presents with a 2-year history of a skin-colored nodule to his lateral finger. The lesion is asymptomatic and he has no trouble opening or closing his hand. It is not increasing in size. He has no other similar lesions elsewhere on his hands or feet. What is the most likely diagnosis?**

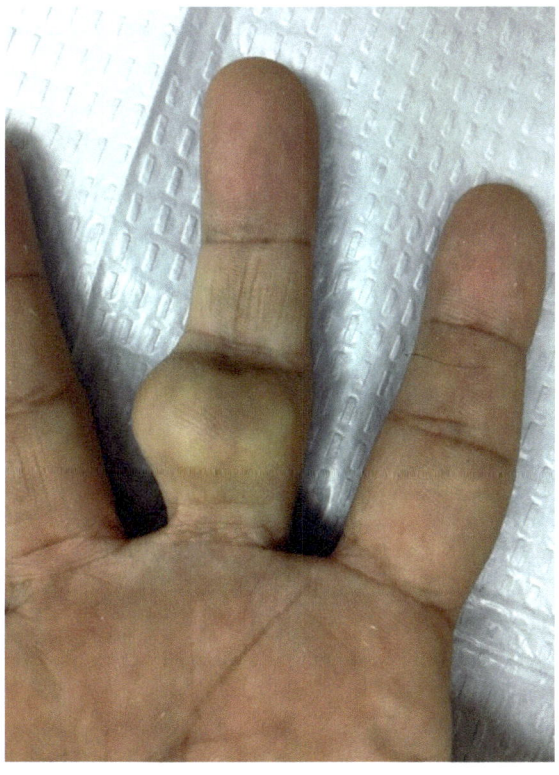

   (a) Endochondroma
   (b) Chondrosarcoma
   (c) Ganglion cyst
   (d) Lipoma

8. **Which of the following statements is the least accurate regarding mycosis fungoides?**
   (a) There is clonal expansion of CD4+ cells that lack the normal T cell antigens like CD7 and/or CD26
   (b) If the patches, papules or plaques cover less than 30% of the total body skin surface, the staging would fall under T1a
   (c) Epidermotropism of abnormal lymphocytes (Pautrier microabscess) is seen typically in the absence of spongiosis on histology
   (d) The 5-year overall survival for patients with non-infiltrating patch lesions (<10% overall skin surface) is similar to the healthy population as these patients often have a good response to topical treatments

9. **Poor prognosis with mycosis fungoides (MF) has been associated with all of the following except:**
   (a) Presence of extracutaneous disease
   (b) Younger age
   (c) Elevated lactate dehydrogenase (LDH) level
   (d) Folliculotropic subtype of MF

10. **What is the least accurate statement regarding Sezary syndrome?**
    (a) It presents often as a diffuse skin rash often involving approximately 80% of total surface area
    (b) It is considered a leukemic phase of cutaneous T cell lymphoma (CTCL) without any bone marrow compromise but involvement of the marrow can be seen in advanced disease
    (c) Pruritus is typically only mild and often localized
    (d) Immmunohistochemical staining typically shows CD3+, CD4+, CD7−, and/or CD26−

11. **Which of following would the most accurate stage in a mycosis fungoides patient who has 25% of the skin surface involved in patches, but no plaques or nodules, no lymph node enlargement, no spread of lymphoma cells to other organs and no Sezary cells in the blood?**
    (a) Stage IA: T1, N0, M0, B0
    (b) Stage IB: T2, N0, M0, B0
    (c) Stage IIA: T2, N1, M0, B0
    (d) Stage IIB: T3, N0, M0, B0

12. **What is the Sezary triad?**
    (a) Erythroderma, generalized lymphadenopathy and atypical circulating lymphocytes (Sezary cells) in the peripheral blood
    (b) Erythroderma, generalized lymphadenopathy, Sezary cells in the peripheral blood with bone marrow compromise
    (c) Intense pruritus, erythroderma, and generalized lymphadenopathy
    (d) Intense pruritus, generalized lymphadenopathy and atypical circulating lymphocytes in the peripheral blood

13. **A 64-year-old otherwise healthy female presents with an enlarging firm erythematous nodule to her umbilicus that is approximately 2.5 cm in size. The patient has reported weight loss and a feeling of fullness to her abdomen for the past 6 months that is worsening. What is the most accurate statement regarding the patient's likely diagnosis?**
    (a) The nodule likely represents a metastatic deposit typically from lymphoma (i.e. non-Hodgkins)
    (b) The presence of this type of nodule is a good prognostic sign
    (c) The nodule is typically a harbinger of an internal malignancy often from an intra-abdominal primary malignancy
    (d) This type of nodule is seen more often in younger patients

14. **A 31-year-old male comes in with a "funny mole" that he states has been present since he was young. He is here for an unrelated rash but he would like the lesion to be evaluated as well. What is most likely the diagnosis?**

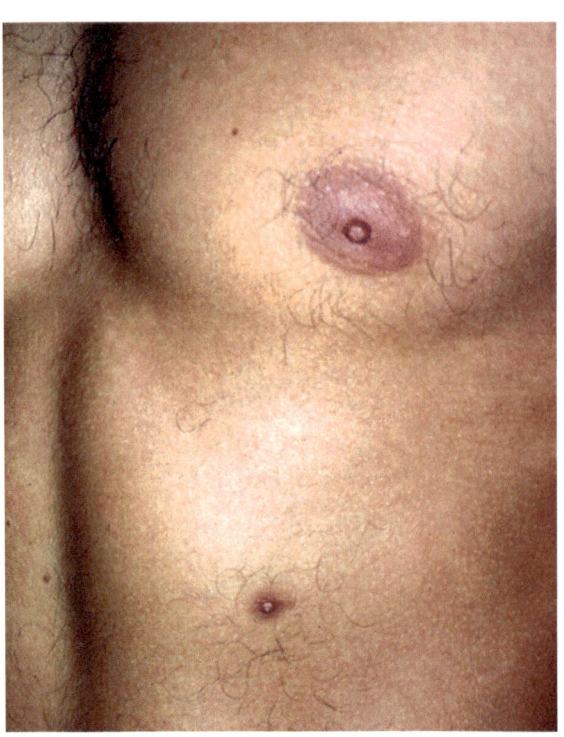

    (a) Congenital nevus
    (b) Becker's nevus
    (c) Hori's nevus
    (d) Supernumerary nipple

15. **Multiple dermatofibromas can be seen in a patient with which of the following?**
    (a) Diabetes mellitus
    (b) Bullous pemphigoid
    (c) Systemic lupus erythematosus
    (d) Lichen planus

16. **The tumor category for melanoma is based on which of the following criteria per the current AJCC staging system?**
    (a) Breslow tumor thickness alone
    (b) Breslow tumor thickness (primary determinant) and ulceration (second determinant)
    (c) Breslow tumor thickness, ulceration and mitotic rate
    (d) Breslow tumor thickness and mitotic rate
    (e) Breslow tumor thickness and angiolymphatic invasion

17. **For a patient with a melanoma of 0.6 mm depth but no evidence of ulceration, regression, perivascular or perineural invasion, or mitoses per histology, would sentinel lymph node biopsy be appropriate?**
    (a) Yes
    (b) No

18. **For a melanoma with 0.3 mm depth, what would be the appropriate wide local excision margin for each side?**
    (a) 1 cm margin
    (b) 2 cm margin
    (c) 0.5 cm margin
    (d) 1.5 cm margin

19. **What is the most common location for melanoma in women?**
    (a) Trunk
    (b) Face
    (c) Legs
    (d) Arms

20. **Which statement below is the most accurate statement regarding desmoplastic melanoma?**
    (a) There is a very low risk for local recurrence after wide local excision
    (b) It stains strongly and diffusely with S100 but negative or only focally positive for other melanoma markers such as HMB45
    (c) It is rarely associated with neurotropism and overall associated with better survival
    (d) Mixed desmoplastic melanoma (versus pure desmoplastic melanoma) appears to be associated with longer disease-free survival

21. **For a patient with a family history of cutaneous melanoma and pancreatic cancer, the mostly likely mutation is:**
    (a) Cyclin-dependent kinase inhibitor 2A (*CDKN2A*)
    (b) Melanocortin-1 receptor (*MC1R*)
    (c) BRCA1-associated protein 1 (*BAP1*)
    (d) Melanocyte inducing transcription factor (*MITF*)

22. **For the angiofibromas shown in the picture, what could be a reasonable topical treatment option from the choices listed below?**

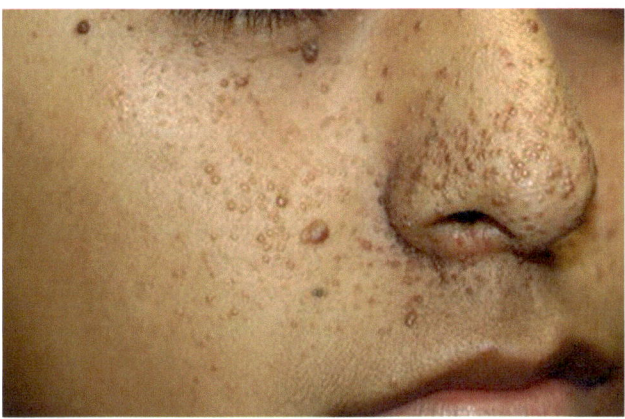

    (a) Topical timolol solution
    (b) Topical roflumilast
    (c) Topical fluocinolone
    (d) Topical rapamycin

23. **Which is the most accurate statement regarding extramammary Paget disease (EMPD)?**
    (a) It is more common in men than women
    (b) The most common location is the vulva
    (c) It typically has an aggressive course
    (d) Paget cells appear eosinophilic on histology and negative for mucin

24. **A 62-year-old postmenopausal female presents with a slow-growing extremely pruritic scaly plaque on the perineal skin involving the vulva. It started as a small itchy papule and then slowly enlarged over the past 3 years. She was diagnosed with lichen simplex chronicus by another dermatologist and was started on a topical superpotent corticosteroid and oral antihistamines, but the patient says this did not help and the rash kept expanding. The most likely diagnosis is:**

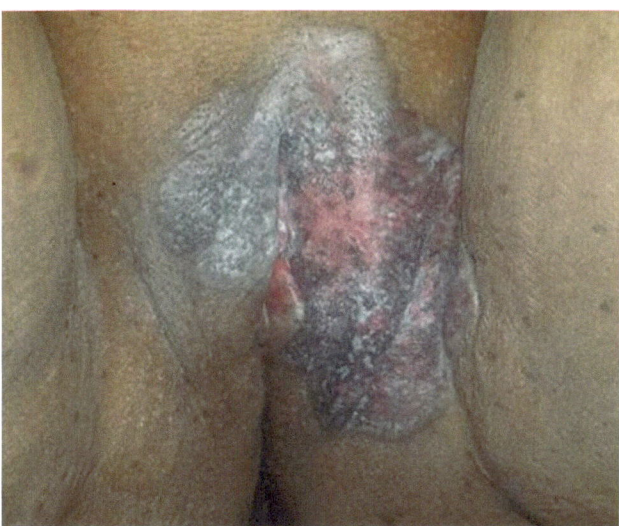

    (a) Lichen sclerosus et atrophicus
    (b) Extramammary Paget disease
    (c) Erosive cicatricial pemphigoid
    (d) Candidiasis

25. **A 45-year-old female presents with a 10-year history of multiple skin lesions that are intermittently painful, especially triggered with cold and pressure. On further questioning, the patient has a history of menstrual irregularities and painful menorrhagia for the past 15 years. Physical examination shows multiple smooth-surface erythematous to brownish papules and nodules grouped on the upper back. Her family history included a sister with similar skin lesions. What would you be concerned about in this patient?**
    (a) Increased risk of renal cell cancer
    (b) Increased risk of medullary thyroid cancer
    (c) Increased risk of pheochromocytoma
    (d) Increased risk of lymphangioleiomyomatosis

26. **The patient in the previous question most likely has a mutation in which of the following:**
    (a) Lysyl hydroxylase
    (b) Laminin 332
    (c) Fumarate hydratase
    (d) Cathepsin C

27. **A 40-year-old male presents with a 1-year history of painless swelling on the left lateral border of his tongue. He states the growth slowly progressed in size over the past year but is now stable. The lesion does not bleed or ulcerate. He denies any preceding trauma or bleeding or ulceration. What is true regarding the diagnosis?**

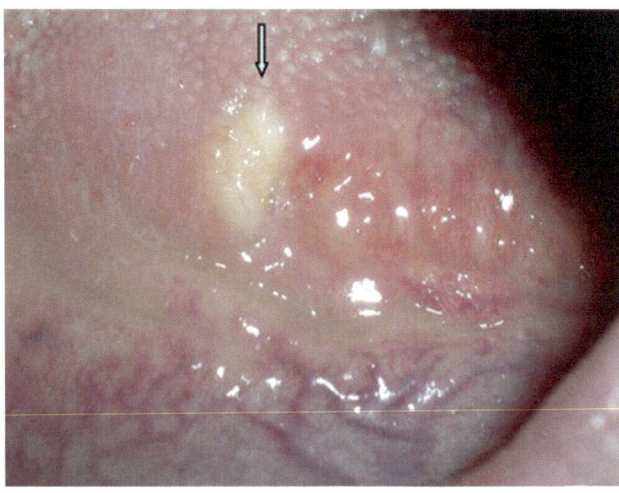

  (a) It is a benign, asymptomatic lesion with a preponderance for the oral cavity
  (b) Histology will show a well-demarcated nodule in dermis consisting of small basophilic round cells
  (c) The treatment of choice for this lesion is wide local excision
  (d) It has a 50% chance of turning malignant

28. **A 33-year-old uncircumscribed male presents with an eroded lesion on the distal glans for the past 6 months. He states he has tried both topical steroid and oral antibiotics in the past without improvement. It has been slowly increasing in size. For the past few months, he has also noticed bleeding and intermittent pain. He has no similar skin lesions on his body. The patient has no past medical history and he denies any joint pain. What is the most accurate statement about this condition?**

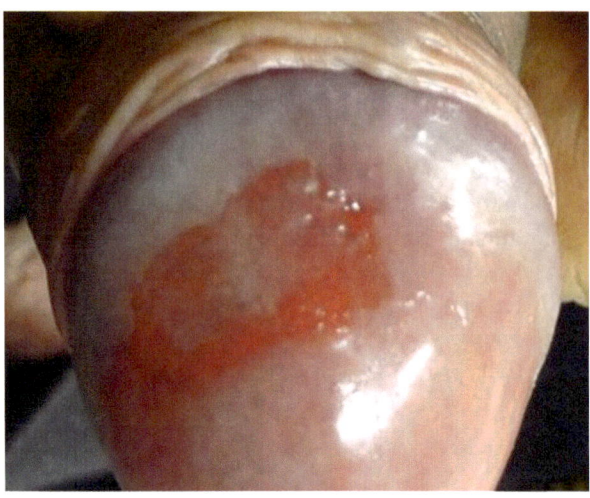

  (a) There is a less than 1% chance of this developing into an invasive squamous cell carcinoma (SCC)
  (b) There is no progression to invasive SCC
  (c) There is close to a 100% chance of progressing to invasive SCC
  (d) There is an estimated 30% chance of developing into invasive SCC

29. **Which of the following is the least accurate statement regarding angiosarcoma?**
  (a) It is a rare but aggressive malignant tumor of vascular endothelial origin
  (b) It is most often seen in elderly males and found on the head or neck
  (c) Predisposing factors include radiation therapy, vascular insufficiency and chronic lymphedema
  (d) It typically has a good prognosis with low rate of recurrence after wide local surgical excision

30. **Which of the following is the least accurate statement regarding Merkel cell carcinoma?**
  (a) It typically stains positive for CAM5.2, AE1/AE3, CK20 but negative for CK7, S100, and vimentin
  (b) At time of diagnosis, there is an approximately 40% chance that the cancer is already metastatic
  (c) It most likely affects young white males between the ages of 20 and 40
  (d) Electron microscopy will show Intracytoplasmic neurosecretory granules

31. **A 22-year-old Asian male presents with a 6-month history of dark red smooth-surfaced papules on his upper arms that are painless. A biopsy shows a wedge-shaped dense dermal infiltrate of lymphoid cells, neutrophils, eosinophils and atypical lymphocytes with epidermotropism. The predominant cell was consistent with CD30+ atypical T cells. What is the most likely course of this disease?**
  (a) It is typically characterized by recurrent, spontaneously regressive papulonodules
  (b) The lesions have 100% chance of turning into lymphoma with time
  (c) The papules are considered a metastatic type of lymphoma
  (d) The lesions will continue to grow and become debilitating

32. **Which of the following favors the diagnosis of a high-risk cutaneous squamous cell carcinoma?**
  (a) Periocular location
  (b) Nasal location
  (c) Perineural invasion on histology
  (d) Features of both basal cell carcinoma and squamous cell carcinoma on histology
  (e) Ulceration

33. **A 17-year-old female presents with multiple asymptomatic cysts on the chest, breast, axilla and inguinal region, sparing only the head and neck, for the past 6 months. The cysts first appeared on the chest and then spread to other areas. On further questioning, the patient states her father has similar lesions as well. On examination, the patient has well-defined and smooth-surfaced small papules and nodules without a punctum and varying in size (2–5 mm). What is the most likely finding if one of these lesions were biopsied?**

(a) The cyst will be lined by stratified squamous epithelium associated with a corrugated eosinophilic cuticle layer, no granular layer, and associated with sebaceous glands

(b) The cyst will be lined by mature squamous cells with a granular layer, no association with sebaceous glands and contain keratinous material and vellus hairs

(c) The cyst will be lined by stratified squamous epithelium with a granular layer and lamellated keratin in the center of the cyst

(d) The cyst will be lined by stratified squamous epithelium without a granular layer and dense, eosinophilic keratin in the center

34. **A 5-year-old boy presents with a painless mass to his neck for the past year that slowly enlarged but is now stable in size. On examination, the mass is mobile and located at the midline of his neck near the hyoid bone. You note that it moves with swallowing. Biopsy shows epithelial lining of squamous or pseudostratified ciliated columnar epithelium and ectopic thyroid gland tissue in the duct wall. Which of the following statements regarding the diagnosis is the most accurate?**

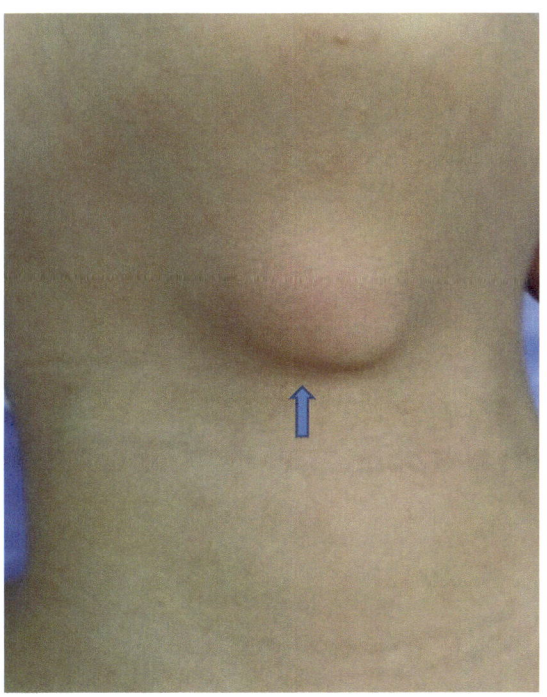

(a) Malignant transformation occurs in near 100% of cases

(b) It can be rarely associated with thyroid cancer (papillary thyroid carcinoma) in less than 1% of cases

(c) Malignant transformation can occur in 30% of cases

(d) It is most often seen in the lateral neck and typically associated with a sinus or fistula

35. **A 66-year-old female presents with a 1-year history of a slowly enlarging lesion to her right chin. The area is painless but has slowly expanded over time. Her biopsy shows small basaloid cells and keratocysts. On higher magnification, cords and strands of basaloid epithelioid cells are seen invading the dermis and subdermis, displaying ductal lumina in a background of hyalinized fibrotic stroma. The neoplastic aggregates show a 'tadpole tail' configuration. What is the most likely diagnosis?**

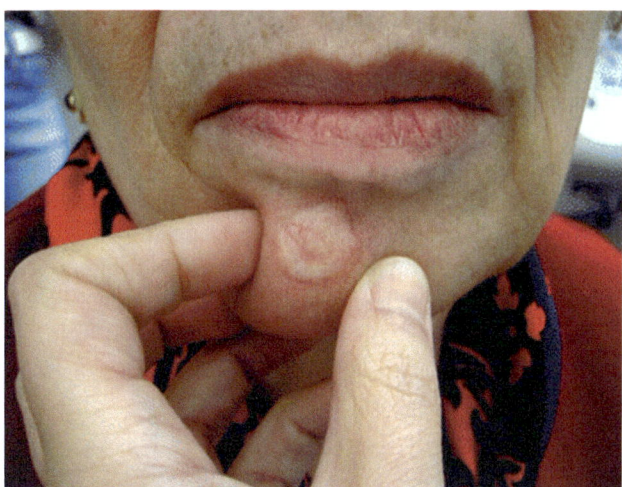

(a) Microcystic adnexal carcinoma

(b) Mucinous carcinoma

(c) Malignant fibrous histiocytoma

(d) Epithelioid sarcoma

36. A 75-year-old male presented with a large translucent cystic nodule filled with watery fluid that had been present for 20 years. There has been no increase in size over the years and the lesion is asymptomatic. Which of the following statement is the most accurate regarding the diagnosis?

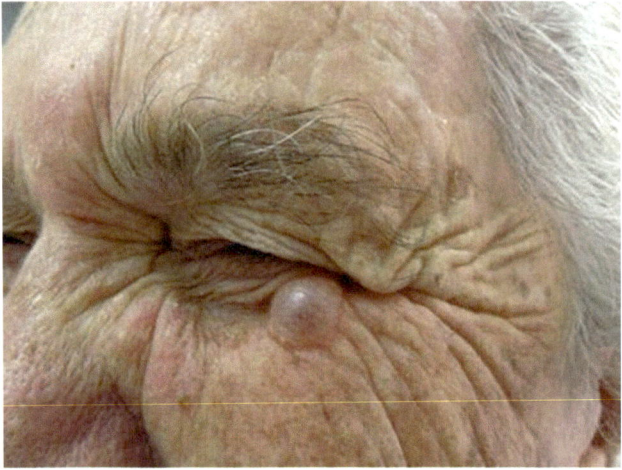

(a) It has the potential for malignant transformation in 10% of cases so excision is always recommended
(b) It often affects vision and can be painful
(c) It typically occurs in adulthood and is benign
(d) It is more often seen in childhood than adulthood

37. A 32-year-old female presents with an asymptomatic nodule of 4 months to the left vulva and comes to you for a second opinion. On examination, there is a well-circumscribed 1 cm red, firm, nontender nodule on the inner aspect of right labia majora. She had a biopsy at a different office and brings her pathology report to you. The report shows a sharply circumscribed dermal-based tumor, no connection to the overlying epidermis, with cystic configuration lined by epithelium and connected elongated tubules and long papillae. The latter has luminal columnar cells with evidence of decapitation secretion. What is the most likely diagnosis?

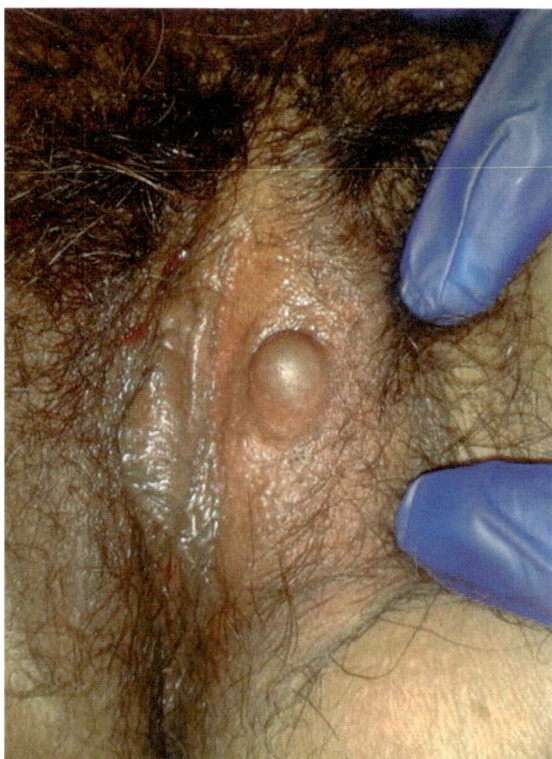

(a) Hidradenoma papilliferum
(b) Syringocystadenoma papilliferum
(c) Epidermal inclusion cyst
(d) Eccrine poroma

38. **A 68-year-old male with no notable past medical history presents with a mobile shiny, nodule lesion for the past 2 years. The histopathologic findings are shown as well in the figure. What is the most likely diagnosis?**

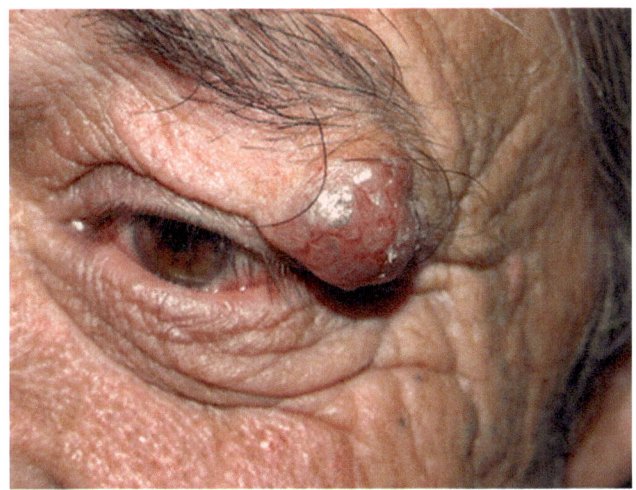

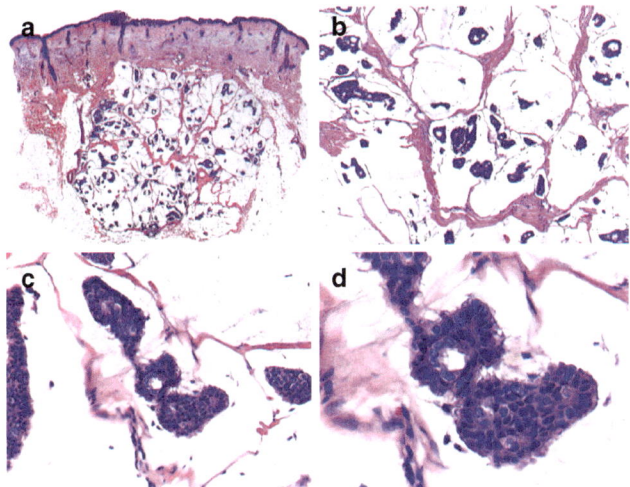

   (a) Mucinous carcinoma
   (b) Syringocystadenoma papilliferum
   (c) Sebaceous carcinoma
   (d) Atypical fibroxanthoma

39. **What is the least accurate statement regarding dermatofibrosarcoma protuberans (DFSP)?**
   (a) It often presents as a slow-growing, firm plaque on the trunk of young adults
   (b) Studies have implicated a chromosomal translocation that results in a fusion protein (COL1A1-PDGFB) that promotes tumor growth through the overproduction of platelet-derived growth factor (PDGF)
   (c) It is an intermediate-grade malignancy with a low likelihood of metastasis but high local recurrence rate
   (d) Wide local excision is always preferred over Mohs micrographic surgery
   (e) Imatinib mesylate, a chemotherapy agent, is currently FDA-approved for adults with an unresectable, recurrent or metastatic DFSP

40. **A 20-year-old female presents with a mass on her left flank for the past 7 months that has been slowly increasing in size. It is occasionally itchy and mildly tender. She has no personal history or family history** of any disease. On exam there is a solitary pink to brown fleshy plaque with central crust measuring 6 × 3 cm. The biopsy is shown in the figure. What is the most likely diagnosis?

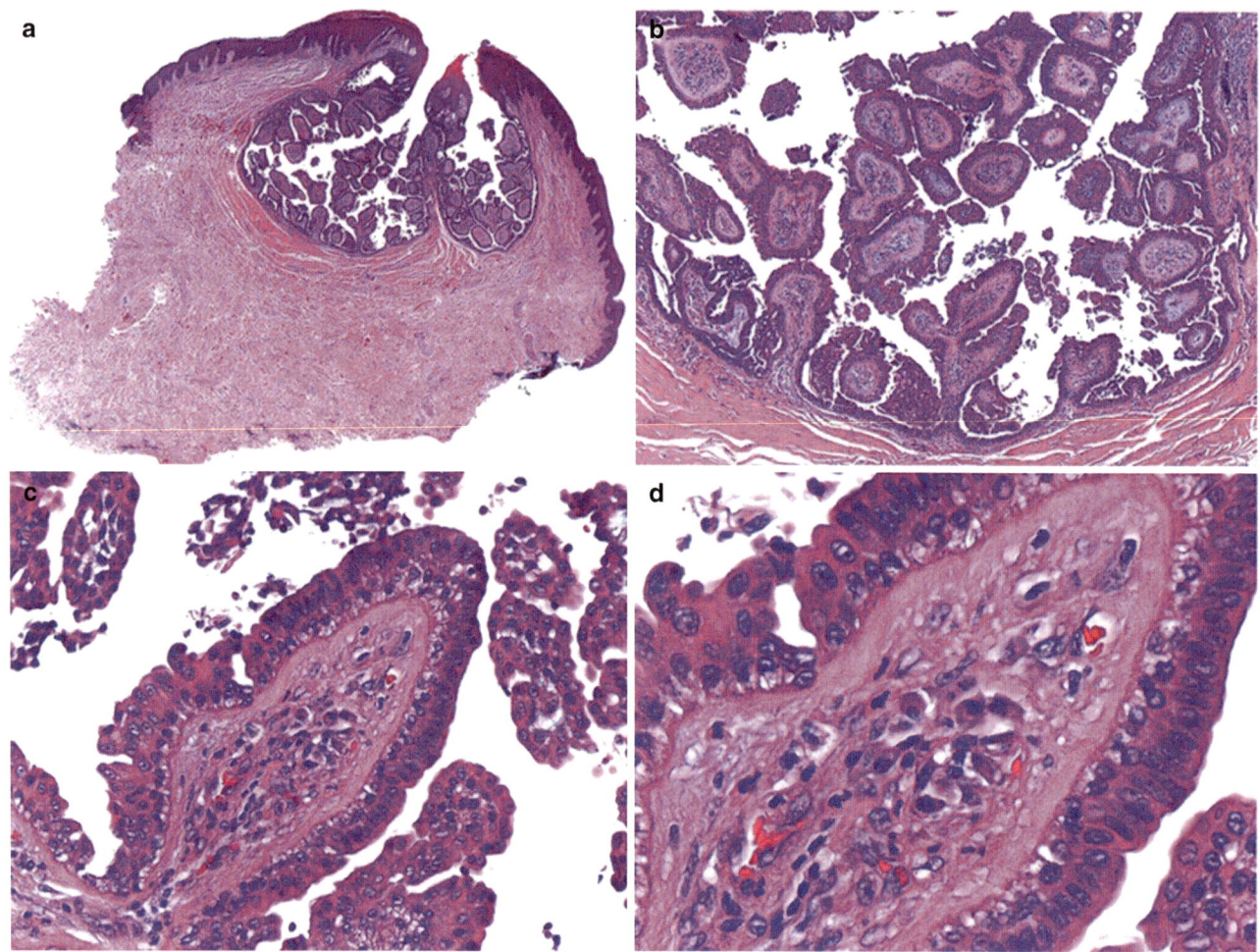

(a) Syringocystadenoma papilliferum
(b) Hidradenoma papilliferum
(c) Verruca vulgaris
(d) Eccrine poroma

41. **An 81-year-old male with a positive history for many basal cell carcinomas to the face and extremities presents for a total body skin examination. He has numerous actinic keratoses but is also found to have a 1 cm erythematous moist nodule on the left upper lateral cheek. The patient had not noticed the nodule until the past few weeks. He denies any pain, pruritus or bleeding. A biopsy revealed a tumor that filled and expanded the dermis and extended to the subcutaneous tissue. Spindle and epithelioid cells with pleomorphism and atypical mitotic figures were also seen. Immunostaining is positive for vimentin but negative for the following: HMB45, cytokeratin A1/A3, CD31, CD34, and desmin with sparse S100 staining. What is the most likely diagnosis?**

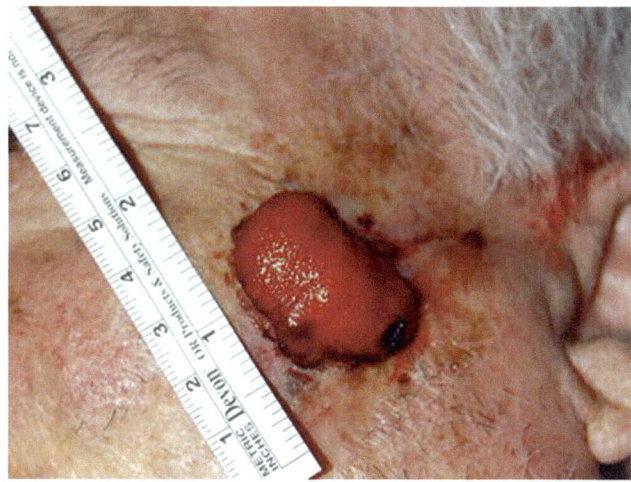

(a) Spindle-cell melanoma (desmoplastic)
(b) Undifferentiated pleomorphic sarcoma
(c) Atypical fibroxanthoma
(d) Spindle-cell squamous cell carcinoma

42. **A 63-year-old female presents to clinic with swelling of her right upper extremity that has worsened over the past 3 years. Her past medical history is significant for stage 3 adenocarcinoma of the right breast, treated 5 years previously with a modified radical mastectomy, axillary lymph node removal and chemotherapy. She developed progressive lymphedema of the right upper limb after this. About 1 year ago, she noticed bruising to her right upper arm that recently turned nodular. She thinks the bruise and lumpiness has spread to her chest, including the site of her prior mastectomy. A biopsy was performed. What is the least accurate statement regarding this patient's diagnosis?**

(a) The biopsy will be positive for CD31, CD34 and factor VIII
(b) Patients most commonly present with pain or discomfort to the affected area
(c) The biopsy will be consistent with a cutaneous angiosarcoma that develops in long-standing chronic lymphedema
(d) This tumor typically presents within 1 year of the development of chronic lymphedema
(e) It often presents as 'spreading bruise' or a raised purple-red papule or plaque that enlarges with infiltration and edema
(f) This tumor can occur in the setting of congenital or hereditary lymphatic malformation or any surgical procedure that disrupts the lymphatic flow

43. **What is the most likely underlying condition in this female patient with the lesions shown on her scalp in the first picture and to the face in the second picture?**

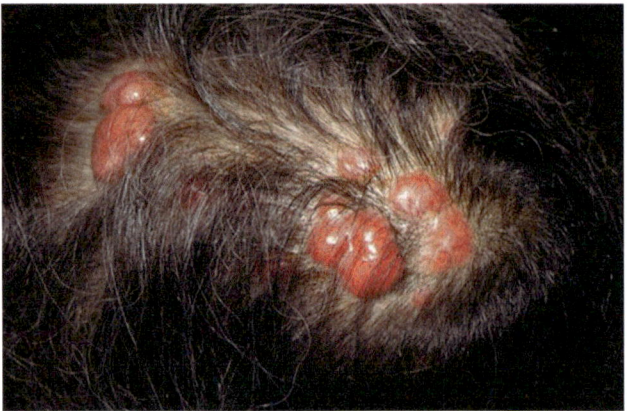

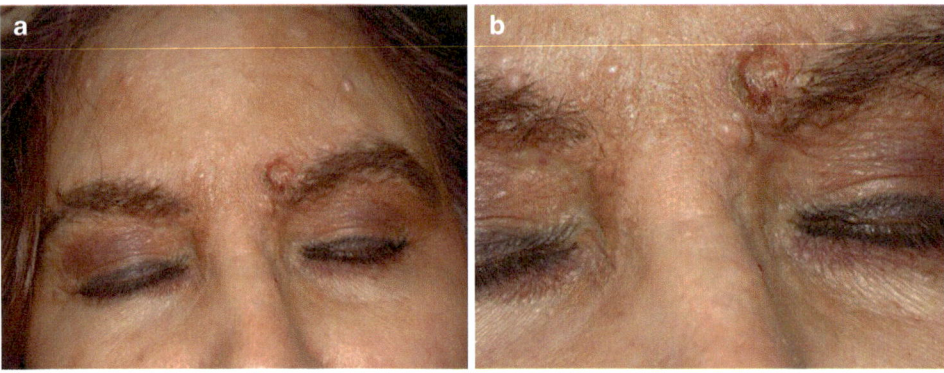

(a) Brooke-Spiegler syndrome
(b) Birt-Hogg-Dubé syndrome
(c) Muir-Torre syndrome
(d) Cowden syndrome

44. **The most likely diagnosis for this dome-shaped, smooth-surfaced papule on the dorsum of the nose with a central pore containing a tuft of fine, white vellus hairs is which of the following?**

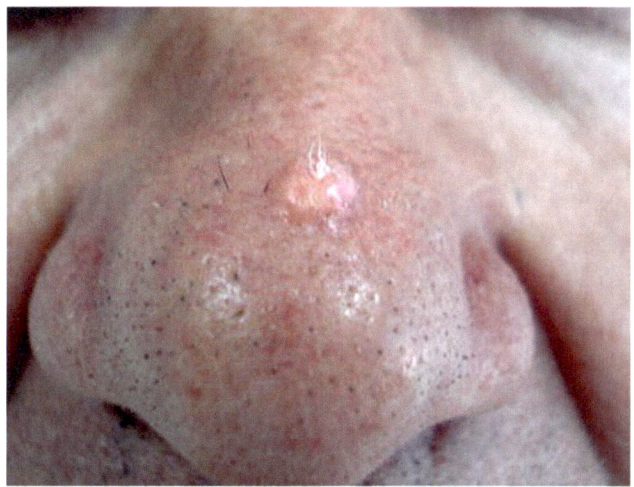

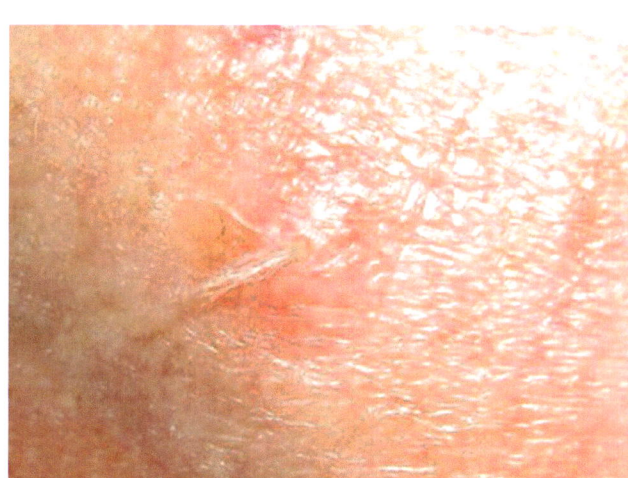

(a) Trichoblastoma
(b) Trichofolliculoma
(c) Fibrofolliculoma
(d) Trichoepithelioma

45. **This young boy has a basal cell carcinoma on his left cheek as shown here. What are possible conditions that can predispose this patient to basal cell carcinomas at a young age?**

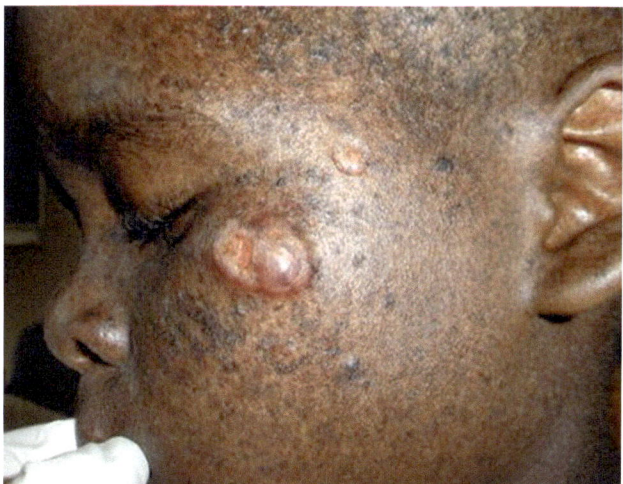

(a) Xeroderma pigmentosum, Gorlin syndrome (nevoid basal cell carcinoma syndrome), Bazex Dupré-Christol syndrome, and Rombo syndrome
(b) Xeroderma pigmentosum, Bazex-Dupré-Christol syndrome, Trichothiodystrophy, Cowden syndrome, and Muir-Torre syndrome
(c) Xeroderma pigmentosum, Gorlin syndrome, Cockayne syndrome, Cowden syndrome, and Muir-Torre syndrome
(d) Xeroderma pigmentosum, Gorlin syndrome, Muir-Torre syndrome, Birt-Hogg-Dubé syndrome, and Rombo syndrome

46. **Which statement is not accurate regarding morphea-form basal cell carcinoma?**

(a) It often appears as a whitish sclerotic plaque with telangiectasias resembling morphea
(b) This variant typically has poorly circumscribed margins and typically extends beyond the clinical apparent limits
(c) The standard of choice for treatment is local excision with the standard margins taken for basal cell carcinoma
(d) It is typically characterized by dense sclerotic stroma, thin epithelial islands and an infiltrative pattern

47. **What is the most accurate statement regarding squamous cell carcinoma (SCC)?**
    (a) Smaller SCCs in sun-exposed areas have a more benign course than SCCs arising in areas of previous trauma (such as radiation site, chronic wound, or scar) that have an increased tendency to metastasize
    (b) There is a higher risk for metastasis in certain locations including the ears, temples and dorsal hands
    (c) Keratin pearls may be seen in poorly differentiated SCCs, while well-differentiated lesions may show little evidence of keratinization and little cytoplasm
    (d) Solid organ transplant recipients, such as renal transplant patients, demonstrate an approximate 20-fold increased risk for invasive cutaneous SCC compared with the general population

48. **Which of the following features of a squamous cell carcinoma would be least likely to prompt treatment with Mohs surgery instead of a wide local excision?**
    (a) Poor histological differentiation
    (b) Breslow thickness ≥2 mm
    (c) Location on the ear
    (d) Ulceration seen histologically

49. **What is the most likely diagnosis of this asymptomatic, exophytic solitary erythematous lesion with a collarette on the sole of the foot with no history of change in the past 3 years? The patient denies any preceding trauma and is on no medications.**

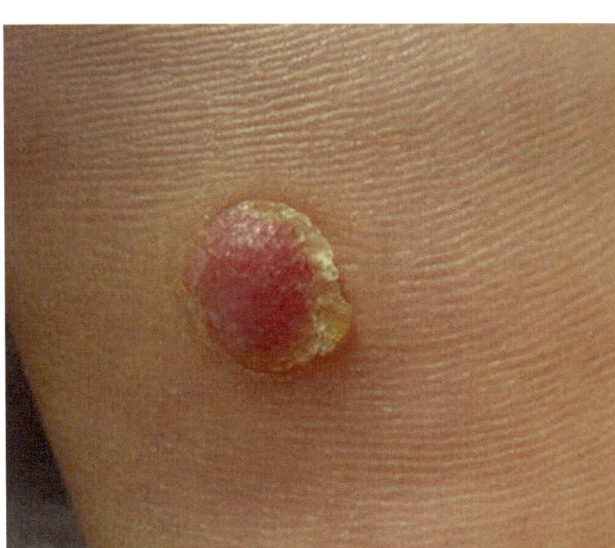

    (a) Pyogenic granuloma
    (b) Eccrine poroma
    (c) Atypical fibroxanthoma
    (d) Merkel cell carcinoma

Answer Key

For further information regarding the below answers, please see Chapter 5 of the corresponding *Dermatology: Illustrated Study Guide and Comprehensive Board Review, 3rd Edition* (2024).

1. **a**
2. **d**
3. **c**
4. **d**
5. **c**
6. **a**
7. **a**
8. **b**
9. **b**
10. **c**
11. **b**
12. **a**
13. **c**
14. **d**
15. **c**
16. **b**
17. **b**
18. **a**
19. **c**
20. **b**
21. **a**
22. **d**
23. **b**
24. **b**
25. **a**
26. **c**
27. **a**
28. **d**
29. **d**
30. **c**
31. **a**
32. **c**
33. **a**
34. **b**
35. **a**
36. **c**
37. **a**
38. **a**
39. **d**
40. **a**
41. **c**
42. **d**
43. **a**
44. **b**
45. **a**

46. **c**
47. **a**
48. **d**
49. **b**

Image Sources

5.1 Phung, T.L., Wright, T.S., Pourciau, C.Y., Smoller, B.R. (2017). Tumors of the Cutaneous Appendages and the Epidermis. In: Pediatric Dermatopathology. Springer, Cham. pp 505–527. https://doi.org/10.1007/978-3-319-44824-4_24

5.2 Requena, L., Sangüeza, O. (2017). Pilomatricoma. In: Cutaneous Adnexal Neoplasms. Springer, Cham. pp 645–669. https://doi.org/10.1007/978-3-319-45704-8_52

5.3 Baykal, C., Yazganoğlu, K.D. (2014). Neural Skin Tumors. In: Clinical Atlas of Skin Tumors. Springer, Berlin, Heidelberg. https://doi.org/10.1007/978-3-642-40938-7_7

5.4 Requena, L., Sangüeza, O. (2017). Inverted Follicular Keratosis and Tricholemmoma. In: Cutaneous Adnexal Neoplasms. Springer, Cham. pp 567–589. https://doi.org/10.1007/978-3-319-45704-8_49

5.14 Requena, L., Sangüeza, O. (2017). Supernumerary Nipple. In: Cutaneous Adnexal Neoplasms. Springer, Cham. https://doi.org/10.1007/978-3-319-45704-8_6

5.22 Phung, T.L., Wright, T.S., Pourciau, C.Y., Smoller, B.R. (2017). Fibrous Proliferations. In: Pediatric Dermatopathology. Springer, Cham. https://doi.org/10.1007/978-3-319-44824-4_25

5.24 Tomar, T.S., Sambasivan, S., Nair, R.P. et al. Extra Mammary Paget's Disease of Vulva—a Case Report. Indian J Surg Oncol 7, 488–490 (2016). https://doi.org/10.1007/s13193-016-0551-z

5.27 Baykal, C., Yazganoğlu, K.D. (2014). Neural Skin Tumors. In: Clinical Atlas of Skin Tumors. Springer, Berlin, Heidelberg. pp 231–243. https://doi.org/10.1007/978-3-642-40938-7_7

5.28 Krasagakis, K. (2015). Erythroplasia of Queyrat. In: Katsambas, A.D., Lotti, T.M., Dessinioti, C., D'Erme, A.M. (eds) European Handbook of Dermatological Treatments. Springer, Berlin, Heidelberg. pp 303–307. https://doi.org/10.1007/978-3-662-45139-7_30

5.34 Al-Salem, A.H. (2020). Thyroglossal Cyst. In: Atlas of Pediatric Surgery. Springer, Cham. pp 29–35. https://doi.org/10.1007/978-3-030-29211-9_6

5.35 Requena, L., Sangüeza, O. (2017). Microcystic Adnexal Carcinoma. In: Cutaneous Adnexal Neoplasms. Springer, Cham. pp 277–299. https://doi.org/10.1007/978-3-319-45704-8_26

5.36 Requena, L., Sangüeza, O. Hidradenoma Papilliferum. In: Cutaneous Adnexal Neoplasms. Cham: Springer; 2017. pp 73–80. https://doi.org/10.1007/978-3-319-45704-8_9

5.38 Requena, L., Sangüeza, O. (2017). Mucinous Carcinoma. In: Cutaneous Adnexal Neoplasms. Springer, Cham. https://doi.org/10.1007/978-3-319-45704-8_29

5.40 Requena, L., Sangüeza, O. (2017). Syringocystadenoma Papilliferum. In: Cutaneous Adnexal Neoplasms. Springer, Cham. pp 55–65. https://doi.org/10.1007/978-3-319-45704-8_7

5.41 Baykal, C., Yazganoğlu, K.D. (2014). Cutaneous Sarcomas. In: Clinical Atlas of Skin Tumors. Springer, Berlin, Heidelberg. pp 359–379. https://doi.org/10.1007/978-3-642-40938-7_13

5.43 Requena, L., Sangüeza, O. (2017). Inherited Syndromes with Cutaneous Adnexal Neoplasms. In: Cutaneous Adnexal Neoplasms. Springer, Cham. https://doi.org/10.1007/978-3-319-45704-8_74. pp 999–1035

5.44 Requena, L., Sangüeza, O. (2017). Trichofolliculoma. In: Cutaneous Adnexal Neoplasms. Springer, Cham. pp 469–482. https://doi.org/10.1007/978-3-319-45704-8_41

5.45 Requena, L., Sangüeza, O. (2017). Basal Cell Carcinoma with Follicular Differentiation. In: Cutaneous Adnexal Neoplasms. Springer, Cham. pp 711–752. https://doi.org/10.1007/978-3-319-45704-8_57

5.49 Requena, L., Sangüeza, O. (2017). Poromas. In: Cutaneous Adnexal Neoplasms. Springer, Cham. pp 177–194. https://doi.org/10.1007/978-3-319-45704-8_16

Dermatologic Surgery and Cosmetics

1. **Which of the following locations would likely give the best outcome if healed by secondary intention?**
   (a) Medial canthus
   (b) Nasal tip
   (c) Malar cheek
   (d) Chin

2. **Which of the following is the biggest concern for an auricular hematoma where blood accumulates between the perichondrium and the cartilage?**
   (a) Disruption of the blood supply of healthy cartilage may lead to necrosis and intractable pain to the ear
   (b) There is no concern as the ear will heal quickly without any sequelae
   (c) The hematoma may mechanically obstruct the blood supply of healthy cartilage and can potentially lead to a "cauliflower" appearance of the ear
   (d) Disruption of the blood supply of healthy cartilage may potentially cause recurrent ear infections

3. **For normal healthy adults, what is the individual maximum recommended dose of lidocaine HCl with epinephrine?**
   (a) 4.5 mg/kg
   (b) 7 mg/kg
   (c) 55 mg/kg
   (d) 6 mg/kg

4. **The most common "adverse" reaction to local anesthesia is which of the following?**
   (a) A reaction to epinephrine that includes tachycardia, anxiety, tremors, and palpitations
   (b) A vasovagal reaction with excess parasympathetic tone consisting of decreased pulse rate and decreased blood pressure with nausea, diaphoresis, and lightheadedness
   (c) Anaphylactic reaction with angioedema and bronchospasm
   (d) A reaction to lidocaine with both circumoral and oral paresthesias and metallic taste

5. **Which of the following anesthetics have the highest risk of cardiac arrhythmia?**
   (a) Bupivicaine
   (b) Tetracaine
   (c) Lidocaine
   (d) Prilocaine

6. **The first symptom typically seen with lidocaine toxicity includes which of the following?**
   (a) Circumoral numbness
   (b) Confusion
   (c) Seizure
   (d) Tinnitus

7. **Which of the following two absorbable sutures last the longest in tissue?**
   (a) Polyglycolic acid (Maxon) and polydioxanone (PDS)
   (b) Polyglactin 910 (Vicryl) and poliglecaprone (Monocryl)
   (c) Polyglycolic acid (Maxon) and poliglecaprone (Monocryl)
   (d) Polyglactin 910 (Vicryl) and polydioxanone (PDS)

8. **Which of the following is the least accurate statement regarding the trapdoor deformity?**
   (a) The deformity often shows an outward bulge of tissue, appearing like a pincushion, with the flap protruding above the surface of the surrounding normal skin
   (b) It is typically due to concentric retraction of a curved scar peripherally and can be seen in transposition flaps
   (c) It typically appears about 3 weeks after surgery, but its appearance may be delayed for up to 6 or even 8 months at times
   (d) This deformity confers a higher risk of necrosis and infection to the site
   (e) It can usually be prevented or minimized by peripheral undermining of the recipient site of the flap to reduce tension and using a flap with the same thickness as the depth of the recipient site

© The Author(s), under exclusive license to Springer Nature Switzerland AG 2024
S. Jain, *Dermatology High-Yield Self-Assessment*, https://doi.org/10.1007/978-3-031-73263-8_6

9. **Which antiseptic is used to prevent surgical infections that may cause deafness if exposed to the inner ear?**
   (a) Chlorhexidine
   (b) Povidone iodine
   (c) Hydrogen peroxide
   (d) Isopropyl alcohol
   (e) Benzalkonium chloride

10. **Unlike the skin of the nasal dorsum and sidewalls, the skin of the lower third of the nose is thick, less elastic, and more sebaceous.**
    (a) True
    (b) False

11. **Cosmetic subunits of the nose include all of the following except:**
    (a) Nasal sidewalls
    (b) Soft triangles
    (c) Nasal alae
    (d) Nasal tip
    (e) Radix (root of nose)

12. **The term "random pattern" in a local flap refers to what specifically?**
    (a) It refers to the blood supply of this type of flap which is not derived from a recognized artery but rather, comes from many unnamed vessels (dermal-subcutaneous microcirculatory plexus)
    (b) It refers to the blood supply coming from a recognized artery that is incorporated into the flap itself
    (c) It refers to vascular detachment of the flap followed by transfer to another region of the body with vascular reattachment
    (d) It refers to isolated perforator vessels supplying blood to the flap from the deep vascular system through the underlying muscle

13. **Which of the following is considered an advancement flap?**
    (a) Subcutaneous island pedicle flap
    (b) Rhombic flap
    (c) Paramedian forehead flap
    (d) Bilobed flap

14. **Which of the following is not considered a local random pattern flap?**
    (a) Advancement flap
    (b) Rotational flap
    (c) Transposition flap
    (d) Axial pattern flap

15. **The scalp should be undermined at the level of the subgaleal space due to its avascular nature.**
    (a) True
    (b) False

16. **The maximum tension site for this flap is at which point?**

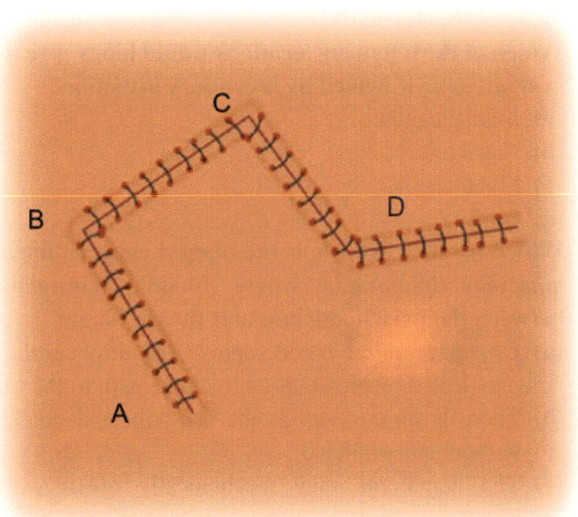

    (a) Point A
    (b) Point B
    (c) Point C
    (d) Point D

17. **Which type of flap is shown here?**

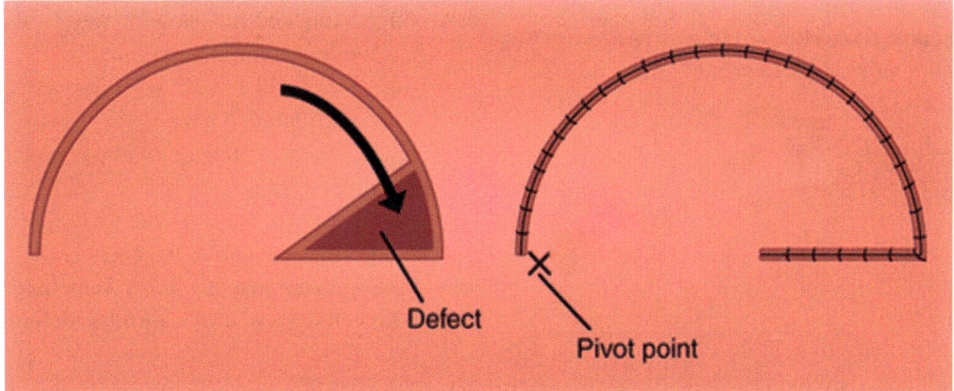

(a) Advancement flap
(b) Rotation flap
(c) Transposition flap

18. **Which of the following is the correct location where the temporal branch of the facial nerve is the most superficial and thus the most vulnerable?**
    (a) Over the bony prominence between the lateral edge of the eyebrow and the ear lobe
    (b) Immediately above the parotid gland
    (c) Approximately 2 cm above the angle of the jaw
    (d) The lateral forehead approximately 2 cm above the lateral two thirds point of the eyebrow

19. **Where is the danger zone for the marginal mandibular branch of the facial nerve?**
    (a) Anterior to the angle of the mandible over the bony prominence
    (b) Immediately superior to the parotid gland
    (c) One centimeter lateral to the tragus
    (d) Upper lateral neck approximately 2 cm inferior to the angle of the mandible

20. **The maximum tensile strength of a surgical scar after 1 year will be approximately what percent of the skin's original strength?**
    (a) 50%
    (b) 80%
    (c) 100%
    (d) 30%

21. **The risk of contracture is more significant in split-thickness skin grafts (STSGs) compared to full thickness skin grafts, and thus STSGs should not be used near free margins.**
    (a) True
    (b) False

22. **Grafts are nourished initially by which of the following?**
    (a) Inosculation in the wound bed
    (b) Imbibition of nutrients in the wound bed
    (c) Revascularization in the wound bed

23. **You are seeing your colleague's patient who had a full thickness skin graft 1 week ago and the patient is very worried as the dressing came off and the area is dark brown and feels hard. The patient denies any pain or discharge to the site and overall feels well. On exam you see a dark purple to black eschar. Which of the following choices is the best next option?**
    (a) Debride the area
    (b) Do nothing as it will serve as a biologic dressing
    (c) Debride the area and inject intralesional triamcinolone to the base to decrease inflammation
    (d) Give the patient oral antibiotics as there is a very high risk of infection

24. **For a full thickness skin graft that is violaceous after 1 week, what color will it most likely be at the 2-week mark?**
    (a) White
    (b) Pink
    (c) Black
    (d) Skin color

25. **What is the primary motion in the flap shown in the figure?**

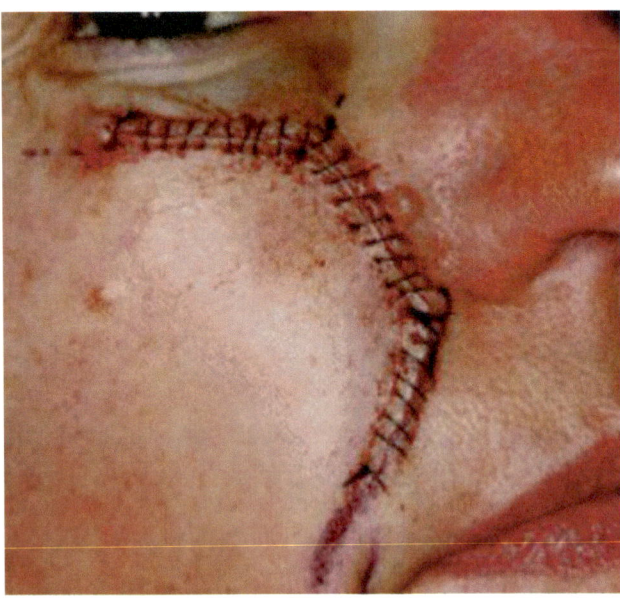

    (a) Advancement
    (b) Rotation
    (c) Transposition

26. **What is the primary motion in the flap shown in the figure?**

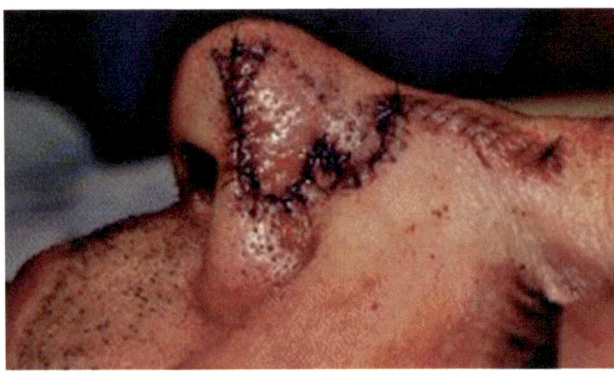

    (a) Advancement
    (b) Rotation
    (c) Transposition

27. **Which of the following statements regarding chronic radiation-induced dermatitis is the least accurate?**
    (a) It typically develops years after treatment
    (b) It often starts within the first 90 days of treatment
    (c) It is typically an irreversible and progressive condition
    (d) May include telangiectasia, hypo and hyperpigmentation, skin atrophy, ulceration, hyperkeratosis, and loss of skin appendages

28. **Antibiotic prophylaxis should be given in which of the following situations?**
    (a) 62-year-old female with mitral valve prolapse with moderate mitral regurgitation
    (b) 62-year-old female with implantable cardioverter-defibrillator (ICD)
    (c) 62-year-old female with a porcine aortic valve replacement
    (d) 62-year-old female with total joint replacement surgery 1 year ago to the knee

29. **Melanocytes are the most sensitive to cryosurgery with cell destruction around which temperature?**
    (a) −5 °C
    (b) −25 °C
    (c) −50 °C
    (d) 5 °C

30. **An M-plasty closure technique is helpful for which of the following reasons?**
    (a) To decrease scar contraction and buckling along scar over a convex surface
    (b) To reduce the length of a scar if it encroaches on an important structure
    (c) To allow for better orientation along curved skin tension lines

31. **Sensory innervation to the earlobe is provided by which of the following nerves?**
    (a) Greater auricular nerve
    (b) Auriculotemporal nerve
    (c) Lesser occipital nerve
    (d) Mandibular nerve

32. **Which of the following supplements is the least likely to carry an increased risk of bleeding?**
    (a) Fish oil
    (b) Garlic
    (c) Gingko
    (d) Ginseng
    (e) Saw palmetto

33. **Damage to the marginal mandibular branch of the facial nerve may result in which of the following?**
    (a) Asymmetric smile
    (b) Ipsilateral eyebrow ptosis
    (c) Pain and swelling to the parotid glad
    (d) Obscuring of the superolateral visual field

34. **Which sensory nerve supplies the skin of the nasal dorsum, tip and supratip?**
    (a) Infratrochlear nerve
    (b) Ciliary nerve, a branch of the nasociliary nerve
    (c) External nasal branch of anterior ethmoidal nerve (latter is a branch of the nasociliary nerve)
    (d) Lacrimal nerve

35. **The patient states she has a crooked smile after getting onabotulinumtoxinA to the lower half of her face. Which muscle would you inject to correct this asymmetry?**

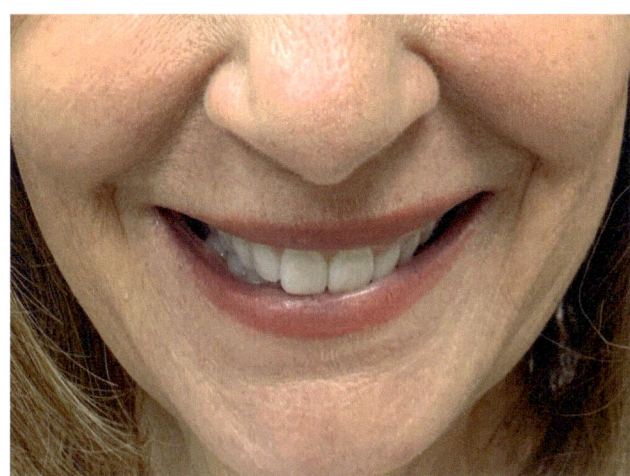

   (a) Right depressor labii inferioris
   (b) Left depressor labii inferioris
   (c) Right depressor anguli oris
   (d) Left depressor anguli oris

36. **A new patient comes for treatment for forehead rhytides. She is not concerned about her glabellar rhytides. When assessing the tone of the frontalis muscle for onabotulinumtoxinA, you ask the patient to sit upright, look forward, and close eyes. If the eyebrows descend toward the cheeks, you should:**
   (a) Proceed to treat both the glabellar complex and forehead lines
   (b) Proceed to treat forehead lines, but do not treat glabellar complex
   (c) Treat the forehead lines first and then treat the glabellar complex in 2 weeks
   (d) Treat the glabellar complex first and then 2 weeks later reevaluate the forehead and possibly lightly treat the forehead lines if possible, being cautious since there is an increased likelihood of brow ptosis

37. **Which of the following is the least accurate statement regarding upper eyelid ptosis due to onabotulinumtoxinA injection to the glabellar complex?**
   (a) Topical apraclonidine 0.5% eye drops can be prescribed to help lift the lid
   (b) Lid ptosis often lasts the entire 12 weeks
   (c) Treatment includes an alpha(can we replace with the symbol for alpha here)-adrenergic receptor agonist that causes contraction of Müller's muscle to elevate the lid by 1–2 mm
   (d) Use digital pressure over the supraorbital rim with the non-injecting hand to reduce risk of diffusion of onabotulinumtoxinA and potential lid ptosis

38. **Which of the following muscles is the most appropriate to inject with onabotulinumtoxinA to help this patient with excessive gingival display or gummy smile?**

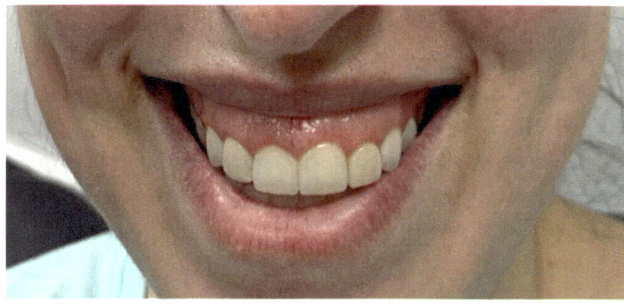

   (a) Risorius
   (b) Zygomaticus minor
   (c) Levator anguli oris
   (d) Levator labii superioris alaeque nasi

39. **What is true regarding the spot size with regard to lasers?**
   (a) When the spot size is decreased, the depth of penetration also decreases due to increased scatter of photons under the tissue surface (more superficial treatment effect)
   (b) When the spot size is increased, the depth of penetration decreases due to more rapid scatter of photons
   (c) The spot size does not affect the depth of penetration
   (d) A general rule is that if you decrease the spot size by half, you will need to deliver half the energy to create similar treatment depth (scatter and decreased intensity of incident beam)

40. **Which of the following is the least accurate regarding lasers?**
   (a) Shorter wavelengths (i.e., ultraviolet and infrared spectrum) have more superficial penetration while longer wavelengths (650–1200 nm) typically have deeper penetration in tissue
   (b) The faster the absorption, the more superficial penetration of the laser
   (c) Power and spot size combined provide power density (how much energy and heat are delivered to the desired target)
   (d) Thermal relaxation time is the unit time for a target to release more than half of the temperature rise in target tissue
   (e) Melanin absorption dominates at lower wavelength, and thus a diode laser is better than a ruby laser for skin of color patients

41. **The chromophore hemoglobin has the following approximate absorption peak(s):**
    (a) 418, 542, and 577 nm
    (b) Broad wavelength between 400 and 1100 nm
    (c) 3000 nm
    (d) 810–1064 nm

42. **Lasers that penetrate deeper into the dermis, such as an Nd:YAG 1064-nm laser, are associated with a decreased risk of epidermal damage and hypopigmentation in patients with Fitzpatrick IV–VI skin types compared to lasers that do not penetrate as deep.**
    (a) True
    (b) False

43. **Which of the following is the least accurate statement regarding tattoos?**
    (a) Professional tattoos are often in the reticular dermis and easier to remove
    (b) The more colorful the tattoo with a multitude of colors, the more difficult it will be to remove
    (c) Amateur tattoos are typically more superficial in the papillary dermis and easier to remove
    (d) The end point of treatment is an immediate ash-white color caused by steam and gas bubbles due to rapid heating of the particles, typically resolving within 30 min following the procedure

44. **Which of the following statements regarding dermal hyaluronic acid filler injection and potential vascular occlusion is not correct?**
    (a) Blanching with a pale, white or dusky appearance may be seen when the vasculature is affected due to reduced blood flow to the affected tissue
    (b) Accidental intra-arterial injection with a filler product in certain locations may lead to obstruction of the central retinal artery and result in blindness
    (c) The supratrochlear and dorsal nasal artery are terminal branches of the ophthalmic artery and filler embolus can potentially flow back to the ophthalmic artery and cause blindness
    (d) In the nasolabial fold and nasal dorsum, the facial, angular, and lateral nasal arteries anastomose with the dorsal nasal artery (branch of the ophthalmic artery) and this area has a lower risk of vascular occlusion

45. **The risk of vascular occlusion is best minimized by all of the following except:**
    (a) A fast injection technique under high pressure
    (b) Aspiration prior to injection
    (c) Use the smallest possible volume to achieve desired affect and avoid overfilling the area
    (d) Avoid bolus injections
    (e) When injecting the glabellar region, injections should be superficial (intradermal)
    (f) Use of blunt-ended cannulas are less likely to penetrate vessel
    (g) Stop injecting if acute pain and blanching seen

Answer Key

For further information regarding the below answers, please see Chapter 6 of the corresponding *Dermatology: Illustrated Study Guide and Comprehensive Board Review, 3rd Edition* (2024).

1. **a**
2. **c**
3. **b**
4. **b**
5. **a**
6. **a**
7. **a**
8. **d**
9. **a**
10. **a**
11. **e**
12. **a**
13. **a**
14. **d**
15. **a**
16. **d**
17. **b**
18. **a**
19. **a**
20. **b**
21. **a**
22. **b**
23. **b**
24. **b**
25. **a**
26. **c**
27. **b**

28. **c**
29. **a**
30. **b**
31. **a**
32. **e**
33. **a**
34. **c**
35. **a**
36. **d**
37. **b**
38. **d**
39. **a**
40. **b**
41. **a**
42. **a**
43. **a**

44. **d**
45. **a**

Image Sources

6.16 Klaassen, M.F., Brown, E., Behan, F. (2018). Transposition Flaps. In: Simply Local Flaps. Springer, Cham. https://doi.org/10.1007/978-3-319-59400-2_8

6.17 Klaassen, M.F., Brown, E., Behan, F. (2018). Rotation Flaps. In: Simply Local Flaps. Springer, Cham. https://doi.org/10.1007/978-3-319-59400-2_6

6.25 Sheehan, J.M., Rohrer, T.E. (2012). Flaps. In: Nouri, K. (eds) Mohs Micrographic Surgery. Springer, London. https://doi.org/10.1007/978-1-4471-2152-7_33

6.26 Sheehan, J.M., Rohrer, T.E. (2012). Flaps. In: Nouri, K. (eds) Mohs Micrographic Surgery. Springer, London. https://doi.org/10.1007/978-1-4471-2152-7_33

1. **Topical dapsone can cause which of the following?**
   (a) Hypothalamic-pituitary-adrenal (HPA) axis suppression
   (b) Methemoglobinemia
   (c) Folliculitis
   (d) Increased risk of herpes simplex virus infection if positive past history of this

2. **Periorbital fat atrophy can be due to which of the following medications?**
   (a) Topical roflumilast
   (b) Topical ruxolitinib
   (c) Topical bimatoprost
   (d) Topical cyclosporine

3. **Methylene blue is the treatment for:**
   (a) Methemoglobinemia
   (b) Calciphylaxis
   (c) Perforating folliculitis
   (d) Agranulocytosis

4. **What is the difference between topical trifarotene and other topical retinoids?**
   (a) Trifarotene is a third-generation retinoid
   (b) It shows selective agonism for retinoic acid receptor (RAR)-γ, the most predominant RAR isotype in the epidermis
   (c) It shows selective agonism for retinoid X receptor (RXR) in comparison to retinoic acid receptor (RAR)
   (d) It shows selective agonism of retinoic acid receptor (RAR)-α, the most predominant RAR isotype in the epidermis

5. **The following are serious but rare adverse effects from isotretinoin except which of the following?**
   (a) Triglyceride-induced pancreatitis if triglycerides are markedly and acutely elevated
   (b) Suicidal ideation or depression
   (c) Trigger of "pseudo-fulminans" if isotretinoin too high
   (d) Increased risk of subacute lupus erythematosus (SCLE)

6. **Which class of antibiotics is the least safe during pregnancy?**
   (a) Penicillins
   (b) Cephalosporins
   (c) Tetracyclines
   (d) Macrolides

7. **What topical acne medication is the safest during pregnancy?**
   (a) Benzoyl peroxide
   (b) Combination of sodium sulfacetamide and sulfur
   (c) Topical retinoid
   (d) Azelaic acid

8. **Which oral antibiotic can cause body fluids (such as urine) to become orange-red in color?**
   (a) Clindamycin
   (b) Rifampin
   (c) Moxifloxacin
   (d) Clofazimine

9. **Which of the following is the most accurate statement regarding oral finasteride?**
   (a) It acts locally by competing with dihydrotestosterone (DHT) for cutaneous androgen receptors
   (b) It inhibits the type 2 enzyme 5-α-reductase and therefore blocks the conversion of testosterone to dihydrotestosterone
   (c) It inhibits both type 1 and 2 enyzme 5-α-reductase and therefore blocks conversion of testosterone to dihydrotestosterone
   (d) It increases the production of hepatic synthesis of sex hormone binding globulin and therefore decreases the circulating levels of androgens

10. **Which of the following is not an accurate statement regarding oral apremilast?**
    (a) Treatment may increase the risk of depression in patients
    (b) The most frequent side effects are gastrointestinal, typically lasting during the first 2 weeks of initiating therapy but often resolving within the first month of treatment
    (c) It is a phosphodiesterase-4 (PDE4) inhibitor and blocks the production of pro-inflammatory cytokines
    (d) Monitoring of labs is essential, including annual screening for latent tuberculosis

11. **Potential side effects of thalidomide include:**
    (a) Somnolence and peripheral neuropathy
    (b) Alopecia, dysgeusia and muscle spasms
    (c) Nephrotoxicity and hypermagnesemia
    (d) Ocular toxicity and hypertension

12. **The mechanism of action for vismodegib is which of the following?**
    (a) It binds and inhibits Smoothened, a transmembrane protein involved in the Hedgehog signaling pathway
    (b) It binds and activates Smoothened, a transmembrane protein involving in the Hedgehog signaling pathway
    (c) It binds the receptor Patched (PTCH1) involved in the Hedgehog signaling pathway
    (d) It binds the Hedgehog protein Gas1 in the Hedgehog signaling pathway

13. **Patients with a thiopurine methyltransferase (TPMT) deficiency treated with a standard dose of azathioprine are at a lower risk for myelosuppression.**
    (a) True
    (b) False

14. **An oral calcineurin inhibitor that suppresses T cell activation and is used to treat psoriasis has the following properties except:**
    (a) Rapid therapeutic action
    (b) Pregnancy category D
    (c) A potential side effect may be gingival hyperplasia
    (d) A potential side effect may be hypertension and nephrotoxicity

15. **Which of the following is a dihydrofolate reductase (DHFR) inhibitor that blocks the synthesis of purines and pyrimidines (nucleic acid synthesis)?**
    (a) Mycophenolate mofetil
    (b) Cyclosporine
    (c) Cyclophosphamide
    (d) Methotrexate

16. **Which medication is a powerful inhibitor of lymphocyte proliferation due to the inhibition of purine synthesis and is associated with a slow clinical response?**
    (a) Mycophenolate mofetil
    (b) Methotrexate
    (c) Hydroxychloroquine
    (d) Cyclosporine

17. **The following are side effects that may be seen with dupilumab:**
    (a) Elevated triglycerides and low-density lipoprotein (LDL)
    (b) Dysgeusia and muscle spasms
    (c) Increased risk of herpes infection and ocular symptoms (conjunctivitis, keratitis)
    (d) Somnolence and peripheral neuropathy

18. **Which two statements below are the least accurate regarding dupilumab?**
    (a) Dupilumab is a human monoclonal antibody inhibiting the α subunit of the IL-4 receptor
    (b) It reduces Th1-mediated inflammation by blocking IL4/IL13
    (c) It reduces Th2-mediated inflammation by blocking IL4/IL13
    (d) Live-attenuated vaccines do not need to be avoided while on dupilumab

19. **What is the minimum age approved for a patient with atopic dermatitis to start dupilumab?**
    (a) 6 years
    (b) 6 months
    (c) 18 years
    (d) 18 months

20. **Which of the following antibiotics at the standard dose would be considered safe to give to a patient with renal failure?**
    (a) Doxycycline
    (b) Ciprofloxacin
    (c) Clarithromycin
    (d) Trimethoprim-sulfamethoxazole

21. **Which is the most accurate order of tetracyclines causing the most photosensitivity to the least?**
    (a) Doxycycline > demeclocycline > minocycline
    (b) Minocycline > doxycycline > demeclocycline
    (c) Doxycycline > minocycline > demeclocycline
    (d) Demeclocycline > doxycycline > minocycline

22. **Which of the following is NOT correct regarding to oral glucocorticoid dosing?**
    (a) A single morning dose decreases the risk of hypothalamic-pituitary-adrenal (HPA) axis suppression
    (b) Divided daily dosing may increase systemic toxicity
    (c) A single evening dose decreases all potential complications
    (d) Alternate day dosing reduces all potential complications except osteoporosis and cataracts

23. **Which is not a correct statement regarding the use of rituximab in the treatment of pemphigus vulgaris?**
    (a) It is an anti-CD20 monoclonal antibody
    (b) It is an anti-CTLA-4 monoclonal antibody
    (c) The effect is thought to be related to B cell depletion
    (d) Rituximab is most effective when given early in the course of the disease

24. **The following statement about ixekizumab is the most accurate?**
    (a) It is a humanized monoclonal antibody the binds interleukin 17A (IL-17A) preventing IL-17A from binding to its receptor
    (b) It is a humanized immunoglobulin (IgG1) monoclonal antibody that binds the p19 subunit of IL-23 and inhibits interaction with the IL-23 receptor
    (c) It is a human monoclonal antibody that binds the p40 protein subunit of both IL-12 and IL-23 and prevents interaction in the cell
    (d) It is a human monoclonal antibody directed at the IL-17 receptor

25. **A 45-year-old male with a history of inflammatory bowel disease (Crohn's disease) has plaque psoriasis with 40% body surface involvement without adequate improvement with oral apremilast, topical corticosteroids and phototherapy. A biologic injectable that would not be a good option for this patient is which of the following?**
    (a) Guselkumab
    (b) Adalimumab
    (c) Ixekizumab
    (d) Risankizumab

26. **A 32-year-old female with a history of relapsing-remitting multiple sclerosis who was treated in the past with pulsed glucocorticoids and dimethyl fumarate presents with 25% body surface involvement of psoriasis with no joint pain. She has tried topical steroids and oral apremilast without significant improvement. She is unable to start phototherapy due to her work schedule. She is not interested in getting pregnant in the future. What injectable biologic would not be a good option to start her on?**
    (a) Adalimumab
    (b) Secukinumab
    (c) Ixekizumab
    (d) Risankizumab

27. **A 45-year-old male with obesity and congestive heart failure presents with plaque psoriasis involving 30% body surface area that includes the genital area and scalp. He has not had a satisfactory response to topical treatment, phototherapy or methotrexate. What injectable biologic would not be a good option for him?**
    (a) Ixekizumab
    (b) Guselkumab
    (c) Adalimumab
    (d) Seckinumab

28. **A biologic injectable that blocks IL-23 for the treatment of psoriasis can be administered less frequently than an IL-17 inhibitor, however it typically has a slower rate of onset compared to an IL-17 blocker.**
    (a) True
    (b) False

29. **Which of the following statements is the most accurate regarding the oral medication tralokinumab?**
    - (a) It is a human IgG4 monoclonal antibody that binds to human IL-13, which in turn prevents IL-13 from binding to its receptor
    - (b) It selectively inhibits JAK1 by inhibiting the adenosine triphosphate (ATP) binding site
    - (c) It is a human IgG4 monoclonal antibody that inhibits IL-4 and IL-13 by binding to the α subunit of the IL-4 receptor
    - (d) It blocks phosphodiesterase-4 (PDE4)

30. **A small oral molecular that selectively inhibits JAK1 by inhibiting the adenosine triphosphate binding site most likely describes which medication?**
    - (a) Abrocitinib
    - (b) Dupilumab
    - (c) Baricitinib
    - (d) Tralokinumab

31. **Which of the following statements about hydroxychloroquine is the least accurate?**
    - (a) Long-term toxicity includes retinopathy, particularly at doses greater than 5 milligrams per kilogram per day
    - (b) The recommendation is for a baseline examination before starting hydroxychloroquine and an annual screening after 5–7 years in non-high-risk patients
    - (c) The risk of ocular toxicity is close to 20% within the first 10 years, even if the dose is less than 5 milligrams per kilogram per day
    - (d) Cutaneous adverse reactions from hydroxychloroquine are typically more common in dermatomyositis than systemic lupus erythematosus

32. **Which of the following are known side effects of the Hedgehog pathway inhibitor drug, vismodegib?**
    - (a) Muscle spasms, alopecia and dysgeusia
    - (b) Somnolence and peripheral neuropathy
    - (c) Nausea, vomiting and diarrhea
    - (d) Hypotension, peripheral edema and tachycardia
    - (e) Sexual dysfunction and depression

33. **Which of the following is NOT accurate regarding the treatment of melanoma?**
    - (a) Ipilimumab (Yervoy) is an anti-CTLA-4 (cytotoxic T-lymphocyte-associated antigen 4) monoclonal antibody that enhances T cell activation against cancer cells
    - (b) Vemurafenib is a highly selective mutant BRAF V600E inhibitor with little effect on wild type BRAF
    - (c) Vemurafenib blocks activation of MAP kinase pathway and this is considered oncogene-directed therapy
    - (d) Approximately 10–20% of melanomas harbor activating BRAF mutations (>90% V600E) that lead to constitutive activation of downstream signaling in the MAP kinase pathway

34. **Elevation of creatinine phosphokinase can be seen with JAK inhibitors but have not been associated with clinical events.**
    - (a) True
    - (b) False

35. **What is the mechanism of action of deucravacitinib?**
    - (a) Tyrosine kinase 2 (TYK2) inhibitor
    - (b) Janus kinase (JAK1 and JAK2) inhibitor
    - (c) JAK1 inhibitor
    - (d) JAK2 inhibitor

36. **Which of the following statement is the least accurate regarding biologic medications?**
    - (a) TNF blockers are broader immunosuppressives compared to IL-17 and IL-23 blockers
    - (b) IL-23 causes upregulation of Th17 cells to make IL-17, so IL-23 blockers are indirectly blocking IL-17
    - (c) IL17A blockers have to be injected more frequently (monthly) to maintain their response
    - (d) Bimekizumab blocks only IL-17F and most likely works better than a biologic with IL-17A inhibition

37. **Which of the following is not true regarding Janus kinase (JAK) inhibitors?**
    - (a) The small size of JAK inhibitors facilitates penetration of the epidermal barrier, thus enabling them to be used in topical formulations
    - (b) They should be used cautiously in patients with increased risk factors for deep vein thrombosis
    - (c) They should be used cautiously in patients with a history of major adverse cardiac events
    - (d) With start of treatment, there is typically a decrease in low-density lipoprotein (LDL) but an increase in the level of triglycerides, so a fasting lipid panel should be checked every 3 months for the first year

38. **First-generation Janus kinase (JAK) inhibitors (i.e. ruxolitinib, baricitinib, tofacitinib) are poorly selective and inhibit various JAKs, whereas second-generation inhibitors (upadicitinib, abrocitinib, deucravacitinib) are more selective and therefore inhibit a narrower range of cytokines.**
    - (a) True
    - (b) False

39. **Which of the following is not correct regarding the medication upadacitinib?**
    - (a) It is a selective JAK1 inhibitor
    - (b) It is an effective treatment for patients with moderate to severe atopic dermatitis or those who have an inadequate response to dupilumab treatment
    - (c) It is FDA approved for atopic dermatitis patients who are 12 years of age or older
    - (d) It is a nonselective JAK inhibitor

40. **A 45-year-old female comes to your office with alopecia totalis and would like to try oral baricitinib. She has no history of cardiac disease or blood clots. The following statements are all accurate about this medication except:**
    (a) A fasting lipid panel should be check at 12 weeks
    (b) It would be reasonable to start at 4 mg daily since the patient has complete scalp hair loss
    (c) If the patient had moderate renal impairment, dose adjustment would be necessary
    (d) Baricitinib is a selective JAK3 inhibitor

41. **If a patient who chronically takes warfarin for atrial fibrillation starts oral ciprofloxacin for hot tub folliculitis, you would most likely expect which of the following change in the INR lab value?**
    (a) Increased INR
    (b) Decreased INR
    (c) No change in INR

42. **The following is a side effect from which of the following medications?**

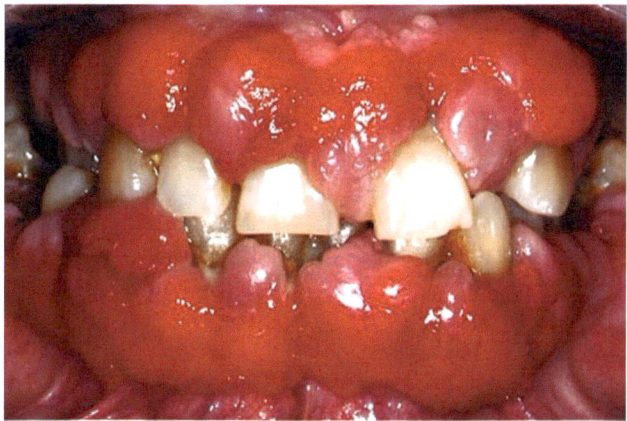

    (a) Methotrexate
    (b) Cyclosporine
    (c) Baricitinib
    (d) Thalidomide

43. **Which of the following medications is the likely cause of the rash seen in the figure?**

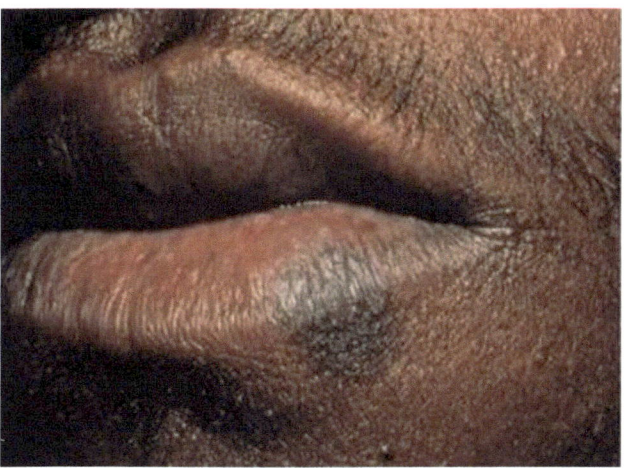

    (a) Naproxen
    (b) Epidermal growth factor receptor inhibitor (EGFRI)
    (c) Hydroxychloroquine
    (d) Hydroxyurea

44. **A 22-year-old female presents with mild fever, lymphadenopathy, and a partially blanching papular rash on her trunk and extremities. She thinks her face appears swollen as well. Her labs show eosinophilia and elevated liver function tests (LFTs). She was recently on a medication for a urinary tract infection but cannot recall the name. When was the medication most likely started?**
    (a) Within 24 h prior to the onset of the rash
    (b) Between 24 h to 1 week prior to the onset of the rash
    (c) Within 2 weeks prior to the onset of the rash
    (d) Between 2 and 6 weeks prior to the onset of the rash
    (e) Between 6 and 12 weeks prior to the onset of the rash

45. **A 43-year-old otherwise healthy African-American man presents for evaluation and management of chronic severe atopic dermatitis diagnosed in childhood. His eczema had previously been mild but persistent. His flares are typically during the winter time and often treated with intramuscular triamcinolone alone. Over the past 12 months he has become concerned as the rashes are more frequent and overall worsening, and he thinks the response to corticosteroid injections only last for a few weeks now instead of months. He also thinks his rash looks different. The patient was given dupilumab at his initial visit and although had significant improvement with pruritus, he only had mild improvement of his dermatitis. Two months later at his follow up visit, he has worsening of his dermatitis and a 10-lb weight loss. What is the next step?**
    (a) Repeat punch biopsy and start patient on abrocitinib
    (b) Start on prednisone along with a steroid-sparing immunosuppressant
    (c) Repeat punch biopsy and order a flow cytometry
    (d) Start deucravacitinib and diagnose his current flare as psoriasis

46. **Oral low-dose minoxidil has the following potential side effects except which of the following?**
    (a) Hypertrichosis
    (b) Bradycardia
    (c) Fluid retention
    (d) Pericardial effusion

47. **What is the potential side effect if isotretinoin is taken concomitantly with an oral antibiotic?**
    (a) Pseudotumor cerebri
    (b) HPA axis suppression
    (c) Methemoglobinemia
    (d) Hyperlipidemia

48. **The least likely medication to cause bullous pemphigoid is which of the following?**
    (a) Furosemide
    (b) Captopril
    (c) Beta-blocker
    (d) Hydroxyurea

49. **Medication-induced acneiform eruptions are most likely to occur with which of the following medications?**
    (a) Erlotinib
    (b) 5-Fluorouracil
    (c) Fludarabine
    (d) Hydroxyurea
    (e) Cyclosporine

50. **Brown discoloration to the gingival third of the teeth is most likely due to which of the following antibiotics?**
    (a) Minocycline
    (b) Flouroquinolone
    (c) Tetracycline
    (d) Doxycycline

51. **A patient presents with this eruption after starting amoxicillin 4 days ago. He feels well and labs are unremarkable. What is the most likely diagnosis?**

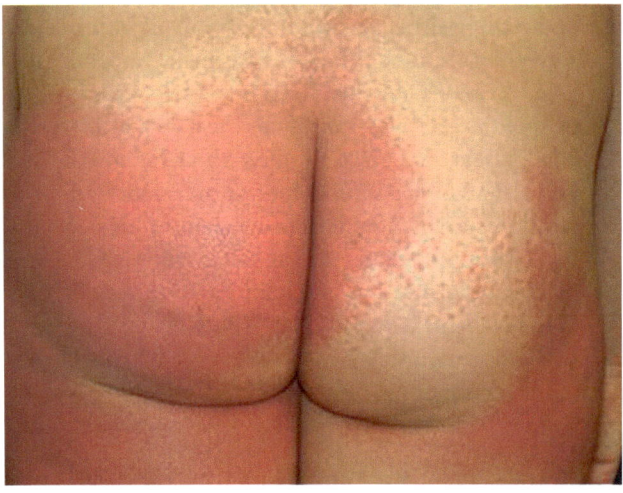

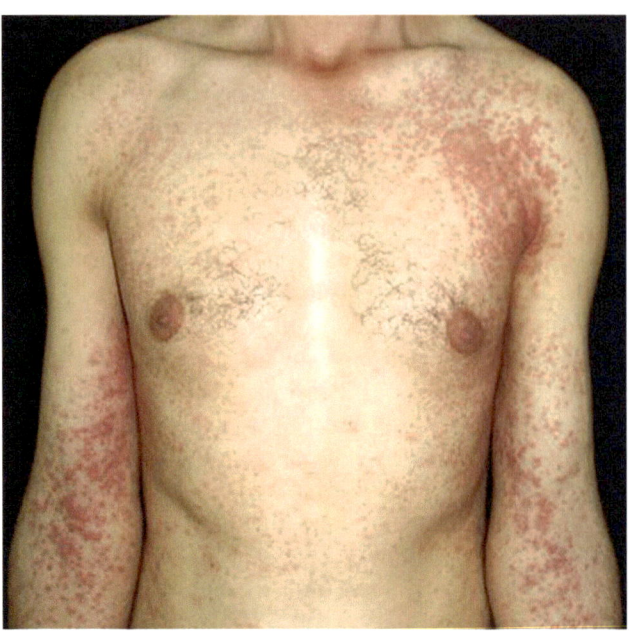

(a) Symmetric and drug-related intertriginous and flexural exanthema (SDRIFE)
(b) Acute and generalized exanthematous pustulosis (AGEP)
(c) Early Steven Johnson Syndrome (SJS)
(d) Drug rash with eosinophilia and systemic symptoms (DRESS)

52. **What is the most likely the cause of this eruption ?**

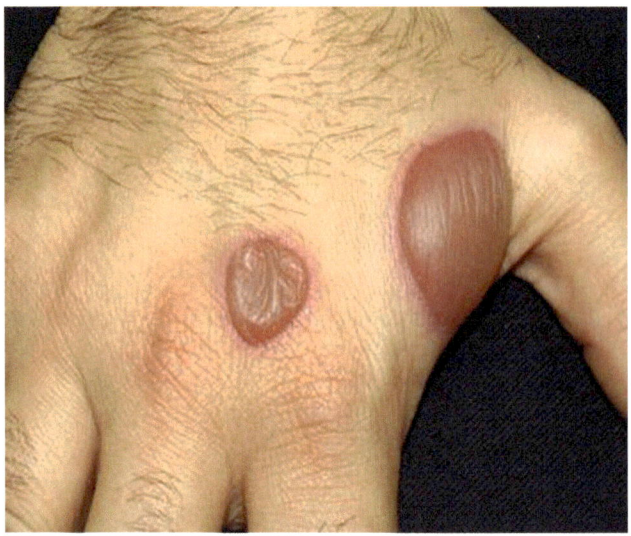

(a) Hydroxyurea
(b) Hydroxychloroquine
(c) Ibuprofen
(d) Acetaminophen

53. **Agranulocytosis is a complication that can sometimes be seen with the use of dapsone. What time frame may this typically be seen after starting the medication?**
    (a) Within the first 24 h
    (b) Within the first 2 weeks
    (c) Within the first 2–12 weeks
    (d) After 6 months of continuous treatment

54. **A patient diagnosed with acute generalized exanthematous pustulosis (AGEP) would have started the culprit medication in what time from?**
    (a) Within 12 h prior to the onset of the rash
    (b) Between 48 h prior to the onset of the rash
    (c) Within 2 weeks prior to the onset of the rash
    (d) Between 2 and 6 weeks prior the onset of the rash

55. **Subacute cutaneous lupus erythematosus (SCLE)-like side effects are most likely to occur with which medication?**
    (a) Minocycline
    (b) Doxycycline
    (c) Tetracycline
    (d) Sarecycline

Answer Key

For further information regarding the below answers, please see Chapter 7 of the corresponding *Dermatology: Illustrated Study Guide and Comprehensive Board Review, 3rd Edition* (2024).

1. **b**
2. **c**
3. **a**
4. **b**
5. **d**
6. **c**
7. **d**
8. **b**
9. **b**
10. **d**
11. **a**
12. **a**
13. **b**
14. **b**
15. **d**
16. **a**
17. **c**
18. **b and d**
19. **b**
20. **a**
21. **d**
22. **c**
23. **b**
24. **a**
25. **c**
26. **a**
27. **c**
28. **a**
29. **a**
30. **a**
31. **c**
32. **a**
33. **d**
34. **a**
35. **a**
36. **d**
37. **d**
38. **a**
39. **d**
40. **d**
41. **a**
42. **b**
43. **a**
44. **d**
45. **c**
46. **b**
47. **a**
48. **d**
49. **a**
50. **c**
51. **a**
52. **c**
53. **c**
54. **b**
55. **a**

Image Sources

7.42 Bontemps, L., Gaultier, F., Anagnostou, F., Ejeil, Al., Dridi, SM. (2021). Drug-Induced Gingival Overgrowth. In: Cousty, S., Laurencin-Dalicieux, S. (eds) Drug-Induced Oral Complications. Springer, Cham. pp 7–24. https://doi.org/10.1007/978-3-030-66973-7_2

7.43 Jain, S. (2017). Pharmacology and Drug Reactions. In: Dermatology. Springer, Cham. https://doi.org/10.1007/978-3-319-47395-6_7. (*Courtesy of* Dr. Paul Getz.)

1. **A 30-year-old healthy female presents with three 1-cm skin-colored firm nodules in a linear fashion to her L ventral forearm for the past 5 month that she noticed after a car accident. The lesions are not enlarging and not painful. She has no medical problems and takes no medications. The biopsy shows a lobular panniculitis. What is the most likely diagnosis?**

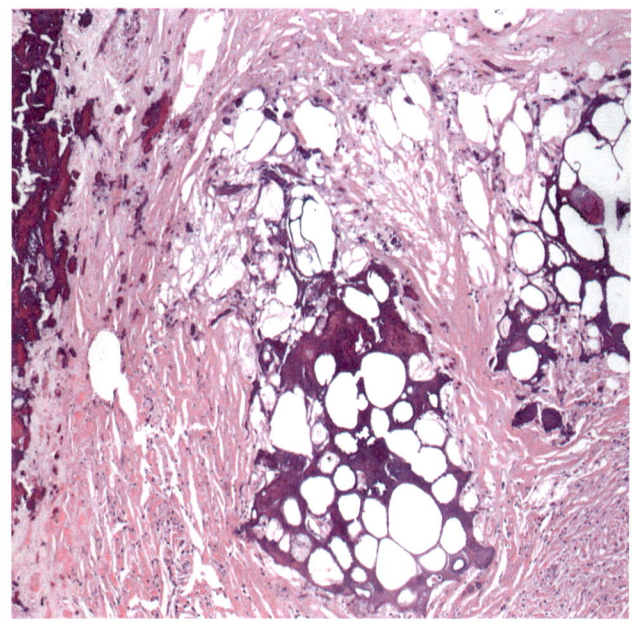

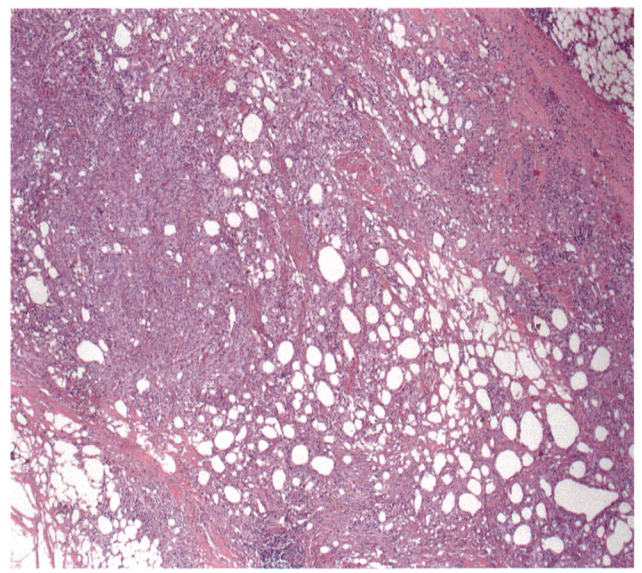

(a) Encapsulated fat necrosis
(b) Sporotrichosis
(c) Lupus panniculitis
(d) Cutaneous calcinosis

© The Author(s), under exclusive license to Springer Nature Switzerland AG 2024
S. Jain, *Dermatology High-Yield Self-Assessment*, https://doi.org/10.1007/978-3-031-73263-8_8

2. **A 73-year-old male presents with a pruritic rash on his trunk and arms for the past 2 months. His past medical history was significant for gastroesophageal reflux disease and hypercholesterolemia. His current medications included atorvastatin, omeprazole and ranitidine and he has started all of these within the past 1 year. He tried betamethasone dipropionate in the recent past but the rash did not improve significantly with this despite using for 4 weeks. A biopsy was taken. What is the most likely diagnosis?**

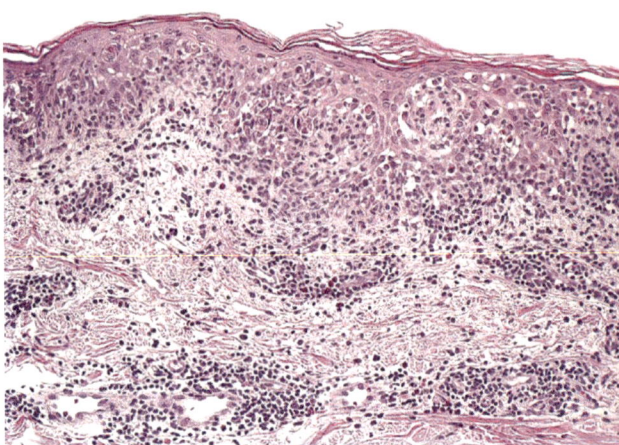

  (a) Syphilis
  (b) Discoid lupus erythematosus
  (c) Lichenoid drug reaction
  (d) Lichen planus

3. **This histologic image is from a biopsy of the vulva of a 9-year-old girl. What is the most likely diagnosis?**

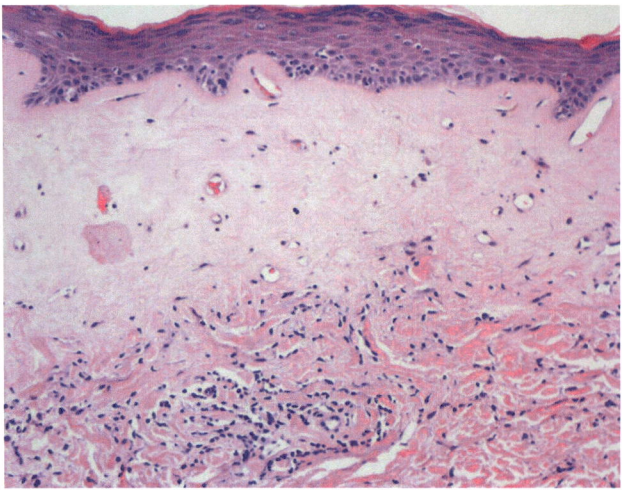

  (a) Vitiligo
  (b) Lichen sclerosus et atrophicus
  (c) Hypopigmented mycosis fungoides
  (d) Contact dermatitis

4. **These histopathology images are most consistent with which diagnosis?**

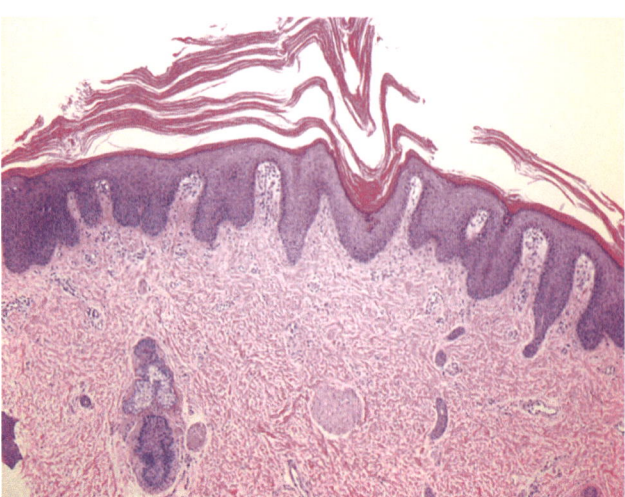

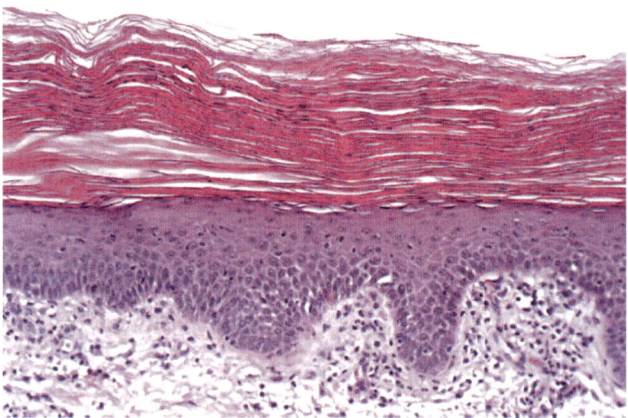

  (a) Psoriasis
  (b) Hypertrophic lupus erythematosus
  (c) Pityriasis rubra pilaris
  (d) Hypertrophic actinic keratosis

5. **A 50-year-old male presents with a 1-year history of an asymptomatic nodule on the face. On exam, there is a red-brown soft 2-cm well-circumscribed plaque on the L mid cheek. A biopsy is shown below showing a grenz zone and a diffuse, polymorphous inflammatory infiltrate including eosinophils. What is the most likely diagnosis?**

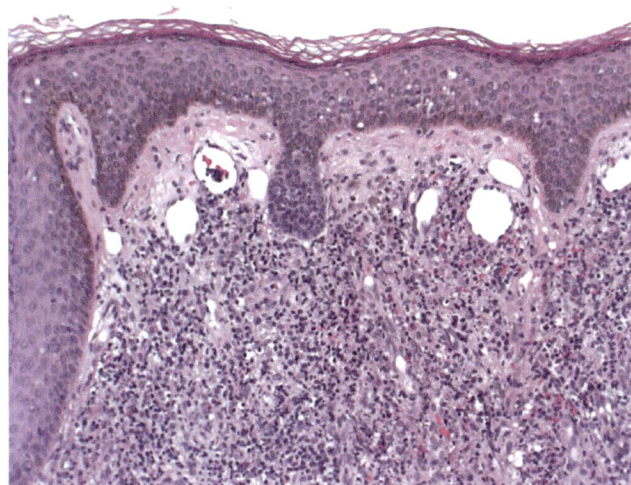

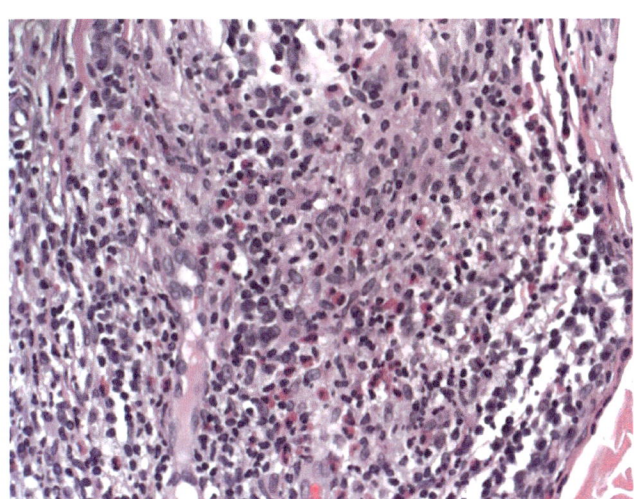

(a) Lepromatous leprosy
(b) Granuloma faciale
(c) Polymorphous light eruption (PMLE)
(d) Leukemia cutis

6. **A 51-year-old female presents with widespread plaques on the face, trunk and extremities over the past 48 h. She also complains of fever, mild sore throat and cough. She has a history of chronic seizure disorder and takes phenytoin for this. On examination, she has several well-demarcated boggy plaques that range from 1 to 15 cm on the back and extremities. The plaques show a target-like appearance with a violaceous center, pale yellow middle zone and a dusky red peripheral rim. The biopsy is shown. What is the most likely diagnosis?**

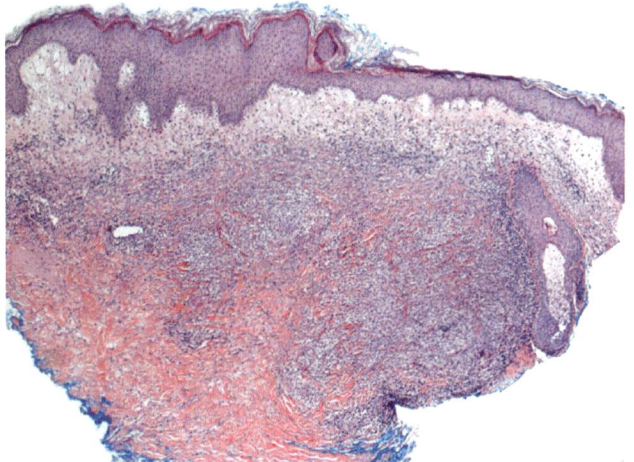

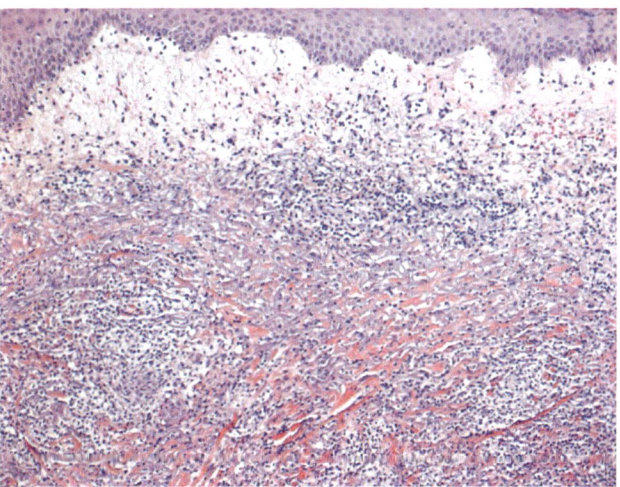

(a) Sweet syndrome
(b) Granuloma faciale
(c) Leukemia cutis
(d) Lymphocytoma cutis
(e) Polymorphous light eruption (PMLE)

7. **A 65-year-old gentleman presents with a 20-lb weight loss and erythematous skin patches and erosions. On further questioning he admits to also having some oral erosions. A biopsy is performed. What will direct immunofluorescence show for this condition?**

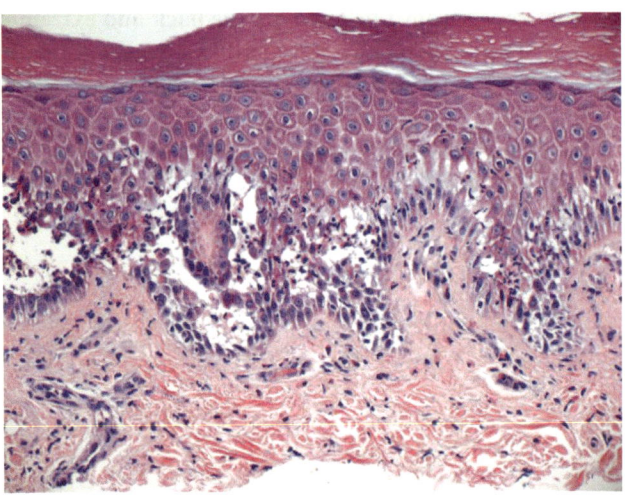

   (a) Deposition of IgG in a linear fashion at the basement membrane
   (b) Granular deposits of IgA in the dermal papillae
   (c) Intercellular IgG deposition in a honeycomb or net-like pattern within the epidermis
   (d) IgG deposits around the vessels in the upper dermis

8. **In the patient above with bullous disease, the most ideal place to biopsy for direct immunofluorescence (DIF) would be which of the following locations?**
   (a) Late vesicle
   (b) Early vesicle
   (c) Erythematous patch
   (d) Normal skin adjacent to vesicle
   (e) Border of erosion

9. **A full-term newborn presents with multiple poorly-demarcated tender firm nodules and plaques on the back with a dusky reddish-purple hue. The biopsy is shown and reveals a lobular panniculitis with an infiltrate of mixed inflammatory cells. What is the most common complication with this condition?**

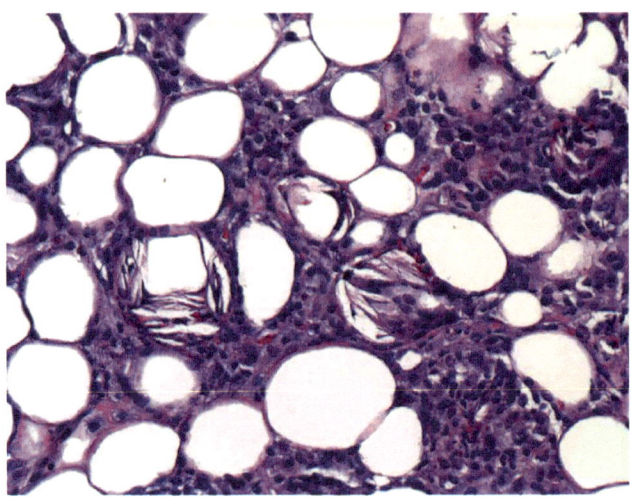

   (a) Hypercalcemia
   (b) Rapid involvement to the whole body potentially rendering immobility
   (c) Congenital heart block
   (d) No complication

10. **A 70-year-old male with no past medical history presents with a 5-year duration of widespread asymptomatic gray pigmentation of the skin and nails. He is not on any medications but he does admit to regularly using a nasal spray for the past 10 years from an online store that he states helps to stimulate his immune system and overall healing. The histologic image from his biopsy shows brown to black granular pigment around the eccrine glands. What is the most likely diagnosis?**

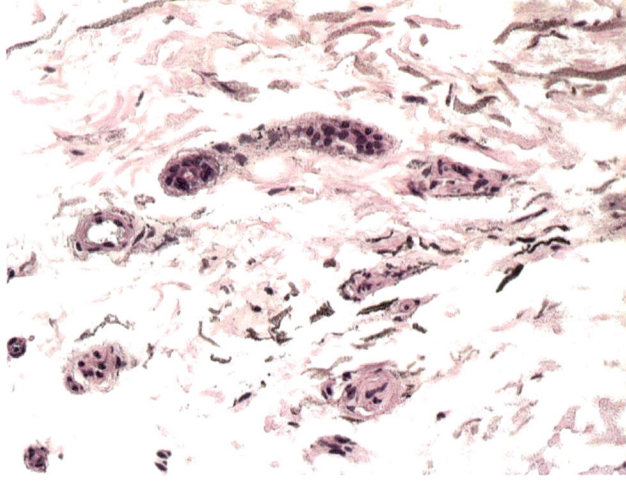

(a) Ochronosis
(b) Amiodarone-induced discoloration
(c) Argyria
(d) Addison disease

11. **What is the characteristic finding seen in the epidermis in this biopsy image?**

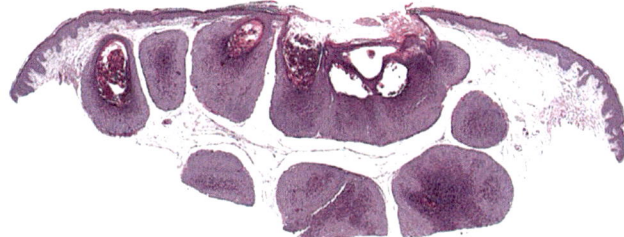

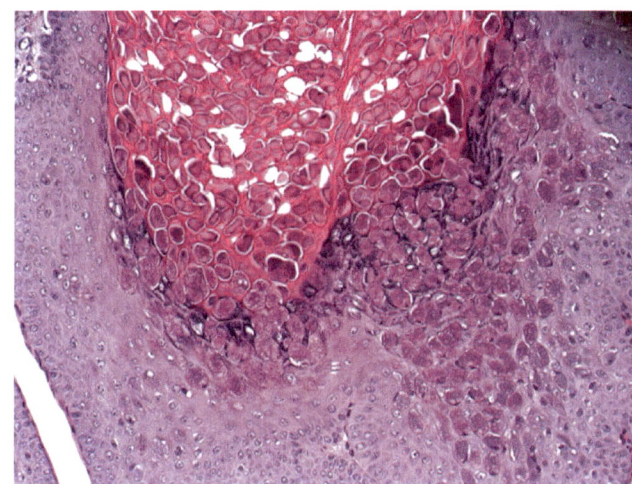

(a) Civatte bodies
(b) Corp ronds
(c) Splendore-Hoeppli phenomenon
(d) Henderson-Paterson bodies

12. **A 25-year-old female presents for evaluation and treatment of acne. During her visit, she also mentions for the past 6 months she has noticed her left third fingernail intermittently throbs. If she accidentally hits or pushes the nail, she feels severe lancinating pain. A biopsy shows the following. Which of the following special stains will most likely be positive in this tumor?**

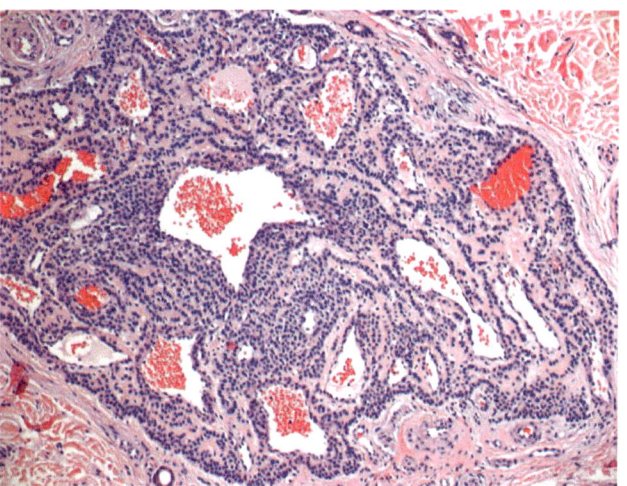

(a) S100
(b) Vimentin
(c) Cytokeratin
(d) Desmin

13. **A 2-year-old-female presents with a 1-year history of a solitary, red to yellow nodule on the scalp. The patient has no medical history and is not bothered by the lesion. The biopsy is shown. Which of the following choices is the least accurate statement regarding this patient's diagnosis?**

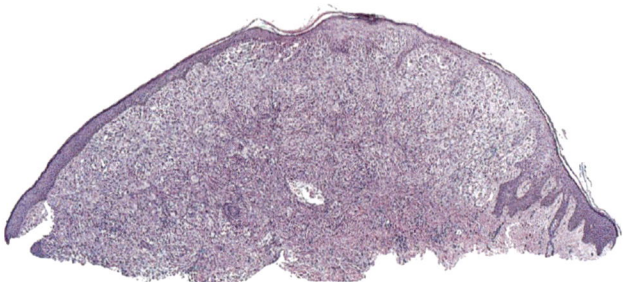

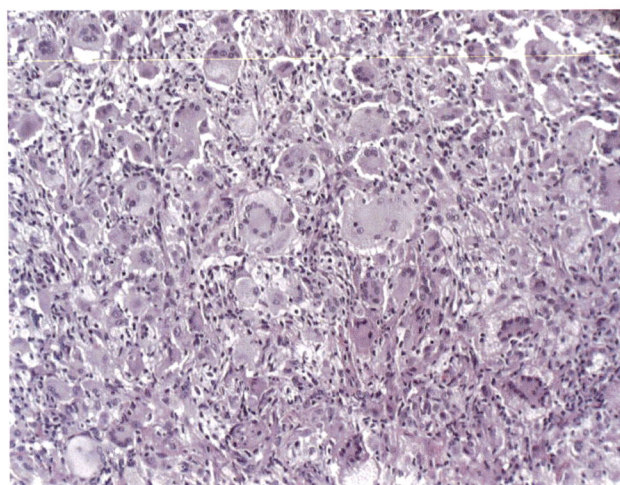

   (a) It is fairly common and often affects infants and young children often in the first 2 years of life
   (b) It is a non-Langerhans cell histiocytosis and the cutaneous lesions usually resolve spontaneously
   (c) In patients with this type of lesion and neurofibromatosis type 1, there is an increased risk of juvenile myelomonocytic leukemia (JMML)
   (d) Cutaneous lesions do not resolve on their own and need to be excised due to their potential for malignant transformation

14. **The ochre-colored banana-shaped bodies are more likely due to which of the following:**

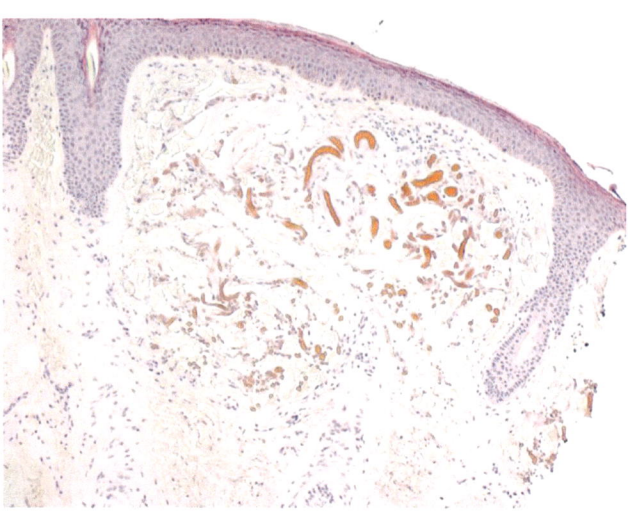

   (a) Hydroquinone
   (b) Silver
   (c) Amiodarone
   (d) Sap from the Japanese lacquer tree

15. **All of the following conditions typically show vacuolar degeneration except:**
   (a) Discoid lupus erythematosus
   (b) Dermatomyositis
   (c) Fixed drug eruption
   (d) Darier disease

16. **Mucin deposition will be seen with all of the following conditions except:**
   (a) Dermatomyositis
   (b) Lupus erythematosus
   (c) Polymorphous light eruption
   (d) Myxoid cyst

17. **A 50-year-old white male presented with a solitary lesion on the right ankle for the past 3 years. On examination, he had a reddish scaly patch with a well-defined ridge-like border. He has lived in Florida for the past 20 years and enjoys being outdoors. He has no other notable skin conditions, except for nummular dermatitis. These images are from his biopsy. What is the most likely diagnosis?**

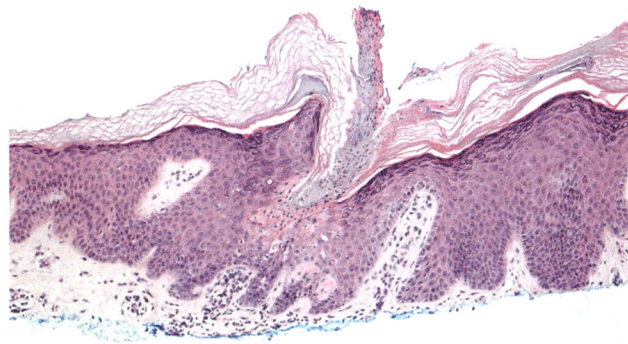

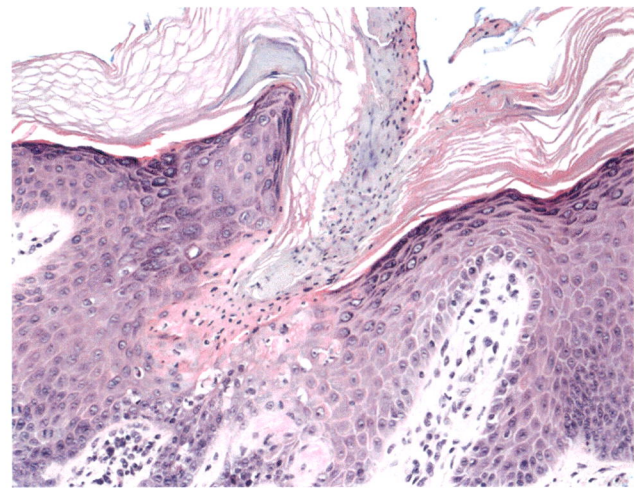

(a) Porokeratosis of Mibelli
(b) Pityriasis rubra pilaris
(c) Nummular eczema
(d) Bowen's disease

18. **Which of the following conditions would necrotic keratinocytes be least likely to see on histology?**
    (a) Erythema multiforme
    (b) Lichenoid drug eruption
    (c) Fixed drug eruption
    (d) Pityriasis lichenoides et varioliformis acuta (PLEVA)
    (e) Granuloma faciale

19. **A small blue tumor with positive staining for S100 but negative for cytokeratin, leukocyte common antigen (LCA) and synaptophysin is most likely which of the following?**
    (a) Merkel cell carcinoma
    (b) Melanoma
    (c) B cell lymphoma
    (d) Sebaceous carcinoma

20. **25-year-old healthy female with no past medical history presents with a subcutaneous nodule on the forearm for the past 6 months. It is not tender at rest but is painful when he presses on the lesion. A magnified image of the histology is shown. What is the most likely diagnosis?**

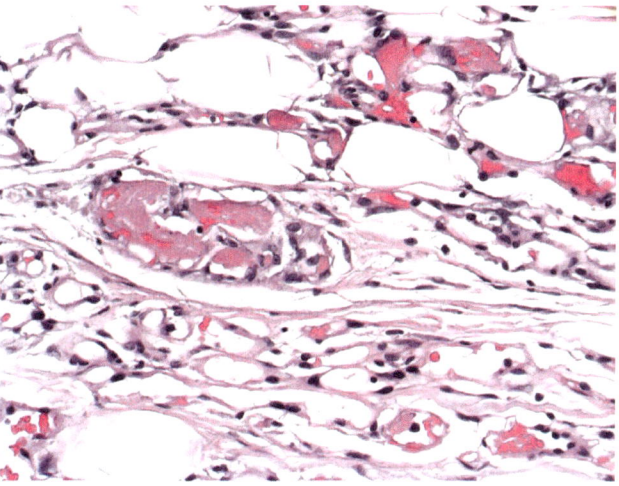

(a) Angiolipoma
(b) Liposarcoma
(c) Cold panniculitis
(d) Tumid lupus

21. **Vimentin staining would be positive in all of the following tumors except:**
    (a) Dermatofibrosarcoma protuberans
    (b) Glomus cell tumor
    (c) Pleiomorphic liposarcoma
    (d) Squamous cell carcinoma

22. **Neuron-specific enolase (NSE) is positive in which of the following conditions?**
    (a) Angiosarcoma
    (b) Granular cell tumor
    (c) Paget's disease
    (d) Leiomyoma

23. **The arrow in the figure is showing:**

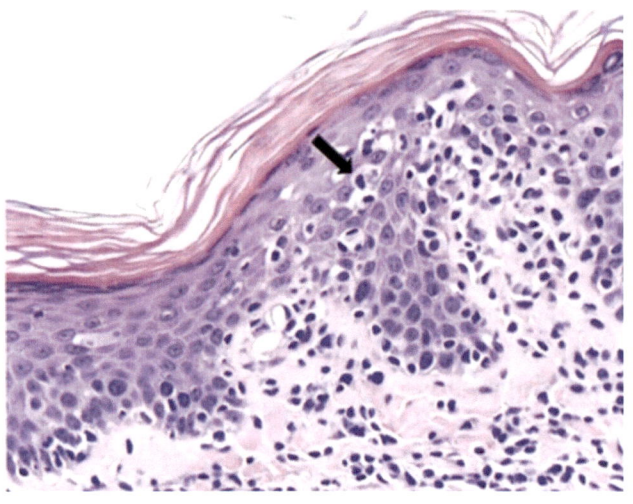

(a) Acantholysis
(b) Civatte body
(c) Epidermotropism
(d) Necrotic keratinocyte

24. **A 35-year-old Hispanic female with no past medical history presents with an annular, indurated erythematous and edematous plaque without any epidermal changes on exam to the face and abdomen. The lesions are tender. The biopsy is consistent with a lymphocytic panniculitis and the following findings in the figure. What is the least accurate statement about this diagnosis?**

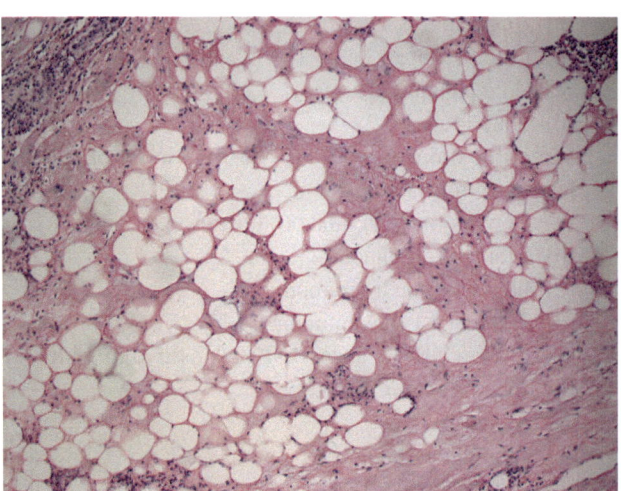

(a) It is a rare variant of chronic cutaneous lupus erythematosus
(b) It typically has a favorable prognosis compared to systemic lupus erythematosus (SLE)
(c) The majority of patients have enough criteria for SLE
(d) Intense inflammation in the fat leads to indurated plaques that can evolve into disfiguring, depressed areas

25. **An 18-year-old female presents with an intermittent pruritic rash to her face, upper chest and arms that lasts about 2 weeks and appears more often during the spring, especially after going to the beach. She does not have the rash now but shows you a picture on her phone. The rash looks like crops of 2 mm erythematous papules clustered together with overall dryness. Her medical history is significant for the patient being a ballet dancer and often takes ibuprofen for muscle aches. Otherwise, she takes no medications. The biopsy is shown. What is the most likely diagnosis?**

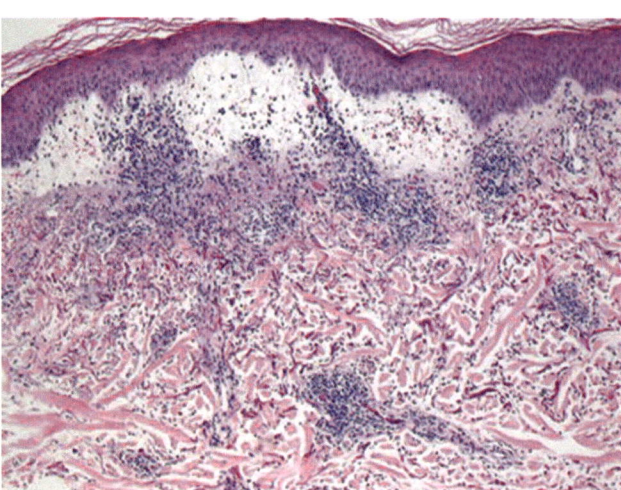

(a) Miliaria
(b) Polymorphous light eruption
(c) Drug-induced photosensitivity
(d) Fixed drug eruption

26. **A biopsy shows thick-walled broad-based budding yeast staining positively for Grocott Methenamine Silver stain (GMS). Which of the following is the most likely diagnosis?**

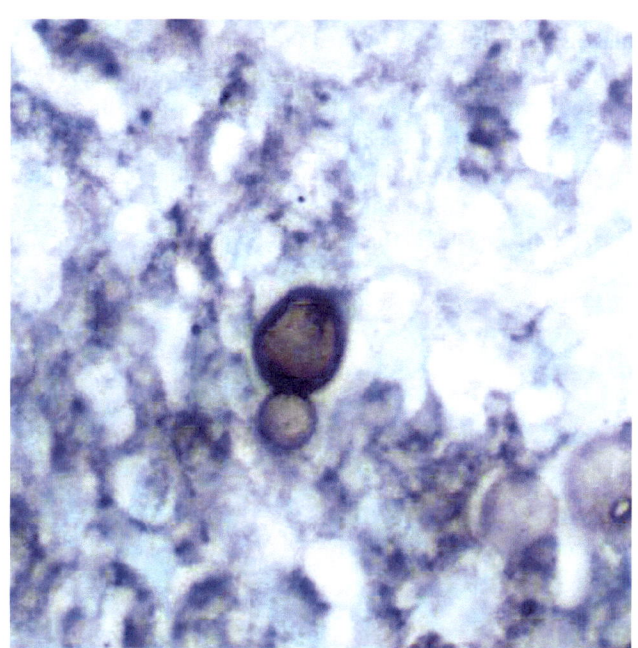

 (a) Blastomycosis
 (b) Lobomycosis
 (c) Paracoccidioidomycosis
 (d) Histoplasmosis

27. **This histologic image is most consistent with which type of infection?**

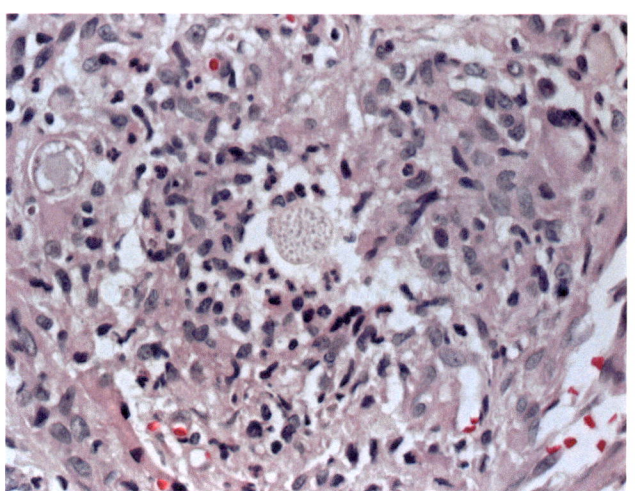

 (a) Blastomycosis
 (b) Lobomycosis
 (c) Coccidioidomycosis
 (d) Paracoccidioidomycosis

28. **A 35-year-old male presents with a tender plaque on his penis for 2 years. His medical history is significant for visiting Mexico two and half years ago and a procedure for penile enlargement. What is the most likely diagnosis with the histology shown?**

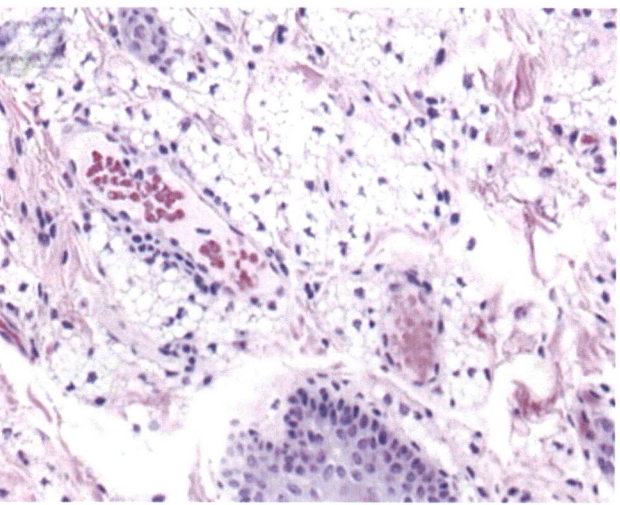

 (a) Suture granuloma
 (b) Paraffinoma or lipogranuloma
 (c) Liposarcoma
 (d) Malakoplakia

29. **A 27-year-old female presented with a red, raised lesion on the left upper chest for the past 5 years that has gradually progressed in size. She has no pain at rest but she complains of pain on palpation. There was no history of preceding trauma to the area and she denies any history of weight loss, fever, chills or night sweats. There is no evidence of regional lymphadenopathy. On examination, a single dark red tender 4 × 3 cm firm nodule with an overlying smooth telangiectatic surface. A biopsy is shown with negative staining for S100. What is the most likely diagnosis?**

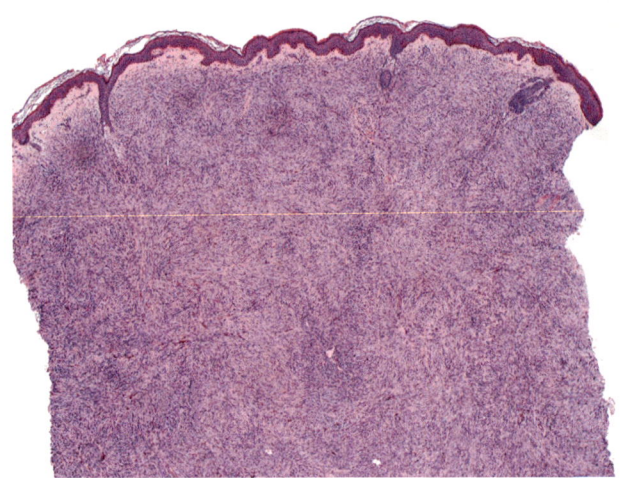

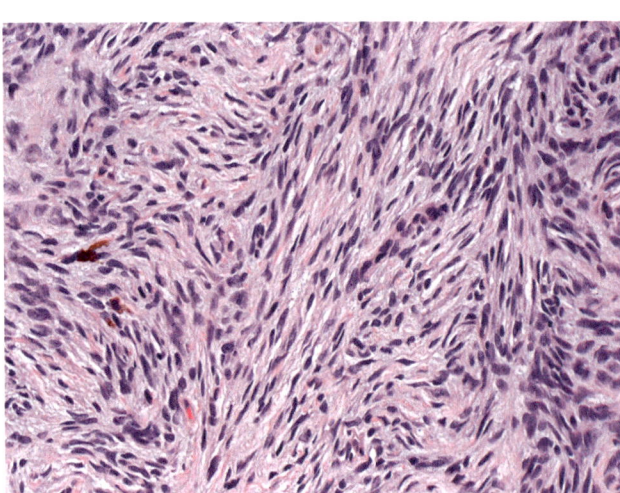

(a) Dermatofibrosarcoma protuberans
(b) Keloid
(c) Leiomyoma
(d) Malignant peripheral nerve sheath tumor

30. **A 33-year-old man with end-stage renal disease of unknown etiology s/p kidney transplantation presents with a 1-week history of a rash over both thighs associated with a severe burning sensation. His history is notable for severe hyperparathyroidism and deep vein thrombosis last year when the patient was hospitalized for a prolonged period of time. Physical exam revealed multiple purpuric macules and papules over the medial aspect of both upper thighs down to the knees. Current medications include oral prednisolone 17.5 mg once daily and oral tacrolimus 2 mg twice daily. His biopsy is shown. What is the most likely diagnosis?**

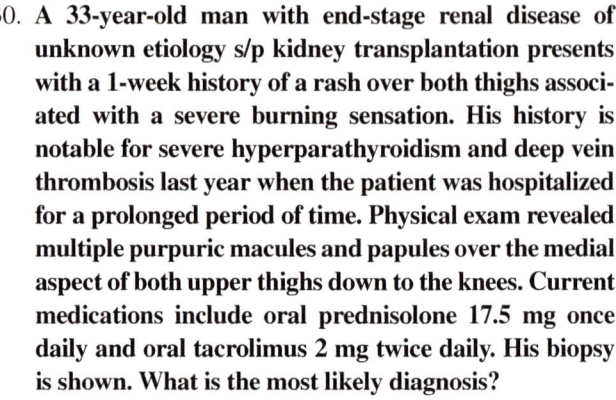

(a) Perforating folliculitis
(b) Calciphylaxis
(c) Nephrogenic systemic fibrosis
(d) Coumadin-induced skin necrosis

31. **What is the most likely diagnosis?**

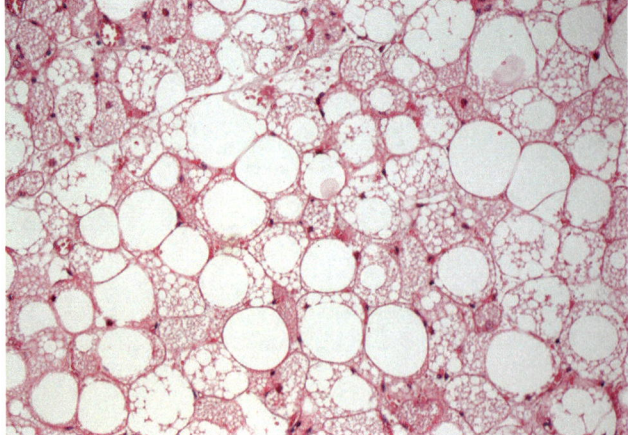

(a) Paraffinoma
(b) Fat necrosis
(c) Xanthoma
(d) Hibernoma

32. **What is the most likely diagnosis from the biopsy shown here?**

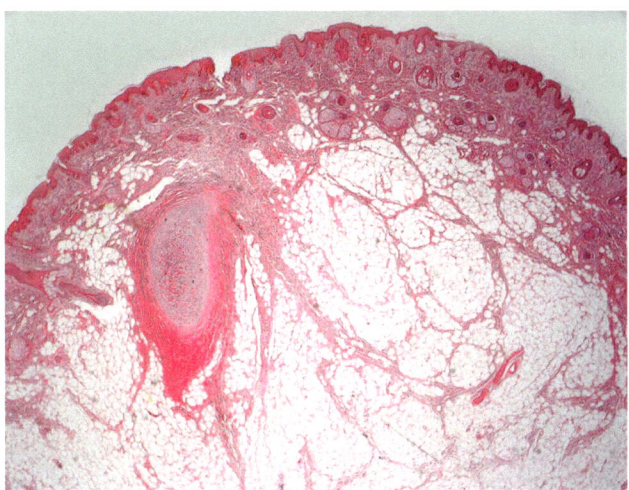

34. **What are the two most common growths that may appear in the figure?**

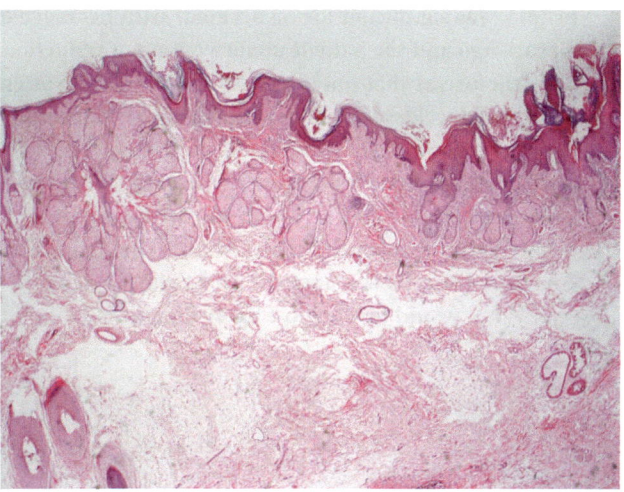

(a) Accessory tragus
(b) Angiolipoma
(c) Nevus lipomatosus
(d) Liposarcoma

33. **All of the following are accurate regarding basal cell carcinomas (BCCs) except:**

(a) In many cases, artifactual retraction of the stroma around tumor islands creates microscopically visible clefts
(b) Morpheaform or infiltrating BCCs can resemble morphea
(c) Morpheaform BCCs are notorious for their subtlety in that the histologic extent often exceeds the clinical impression, leading to high recurrence rates after standard excision
(d) Nodular BCCs are usually more aggressive than morpheaform BCCs
(e) All subtypes of BCC share in common the presence of aggregations of basaloid keratinocytes surrounded by stromal tissue with typical connection to the epidermis, and tumor aggregates may demonstrate peripheral palisading of nuclei

(a) Trichoblastoma and syringocystadenoma papilliferum
(b) Basal cell carcinoma and trichoblastoma
(c) Syringocystadenoma papilliferum and basal cell carcinoma
(d) Trichoepithelioma and trichoblastoma

35. **A 49-year-old male presents with a palpable skin-colored nodule to the right cheek for the past 2 years. Exam shows a firm but nontender nodule. Medical history was significant for an accident with his bicycle 3 years ago and the patient underwent open reduction of a fracture at that time. He noticed the nodule after the bicycle accident and it has slowly grown since. This figure shows a magnified image of the biopsy. The cells were positive for cytokeratin-7, gross cystic disease fluid protein (GCDFP) 15 and mucin 1 protein but negative for cytokeratin 20 (CK20). The fluid surrounding the cells was periodic acid-Schiff (PAS) positive. What would be the most likely diagnosis?**

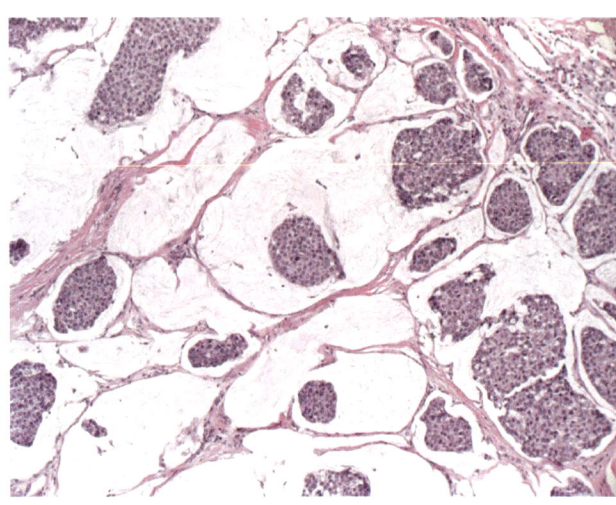

(a) Pleiomorphic liposarcoma
(b) Chondroid lipoma
(c) Primary mucinous carcinoma
(d) Hibernoma

36. **A biopsy from a blister shows a subepidermal bulla with eccrine gland necrosis. What is the most likely etiology of the blister?**
    (a) Coma
    (b) Acute trauma
    (c) Diabetes
    (d) Constant friction

Answer Key
1. **a**
2. **c**
3. **b**
4. **c**
5. **b**
6. **a**
7. **c**
8. **d**
9. **a**
10. **c**
11. **d**
12. **b**
13. **d**
14. **a**
15. **d**
16. **c**
17. **a**
18. **e**
19. **b**
20. **a**
21. **d**
22. **b**
23. **c**
24. **c**
25. **b**
26. **a**
27. **c**
28. **b**
29. **a**
30. **b**
31. **d**
32. **a**
33. **d**
34. **a**
35. **c**
36. **a**

Image Sources

8.1 Phung, T.L., Wright, T.S., Pourciau, C.Y., Smoller, B.R. (2017). Panniculitis. In: Pediatric Dermatopathology. Springer, Cham. pp 197–208. https://doi.org/10.1007/978-3-319-44824-4_9

8.2 Cockerell, C., Mihm, M.C., Hall, B.J., Chisholm, C., Jessup, C., Merola, M. (2014). Interface (Lichenoid) Dermatoses. In: Dermatopathology. Springer, London. pp 3–14. https://doi.org/10.1007/978-1-4471-5448-8_1

8.3 Phung, T.L., Wright, T.S., Pourciau, C.Y., Smoller, B.R. (2017). Interface Dermatoses. In: Pediatric Dermatopathology. Springer, Cham. pp 87–120. https://doi.org/10.1007/978-3-319-44824-4_4

8.4 **a**, Phung, T.L., Wright, T.S., Pourciau, C.Y., Smoller, B.R. (2017). Papulosquamous Diseases. In: Pediatric Dermatopathology. Springer, Cham. https://doi.org/10.1007/978-3-319-44824-4_2. **b**, Cockerell, C., Mihm, M.C., Hall, B.J., Chisholm, C., Jessup, C., Merola, M. (2014). Psoriasiform Dermatoses. In: Dermatopathology. Springer, London. pp 33–41. https://doi.org/10.1007/978-1-4471-5448-8_3

8.5 Cockerell, C., Mihm, M.C., Hall, B.J., Chisholm, C., Jessup, C., Merola, M. (2014). Vasculitic and Vasculopathic Disorders. In: Dermatopathology. pp 67–93. Springer, London. https://doi.org/10.1007/978-1-4471-5448-8_5

8.6 Cockerell, C., Mihm, M.C., Hall, B.J., Chisholm, C., Jessup, C., Merola, M. (2014). Vasculitic and Vasculopathic Disorders. In: Dermatopathology. pp 67–93. Springer, London. https://doi.org/10.1007/978-1-4471-5448-8_5

8.7 Cockerell, C., Mihm, M.C., Hall, B.J., Chisholm, C., Jessup, C., Merola, M. (2014). Vesiculobullous Diseases. In: Dermatopathology. Springer, London. pp 43–65. https://doi.org/10.1007/978-1-4471-5448-8_4

8.9 Cockerell, C., Mihm, M.C., Hall, B.J., Chisholm, C., Jessup, C., Merola, M. (2014). Panniculitides. In: Dermatopathology. Springer, London. pp 113–125. https://doi.org/10.1007/978-1-4471-5448-8_7

8.10 Cockerell, C., Mihm, M.C., Hall, B.J., Chisholm, C., Jessup, C., Merola, M. (2014). Drug Reaction Patterns. In: Dermatopathology. Springer, London. pp 185–200. https://doi.org/10.1007/978-1-4471-5448-8_14

8.11 Cockerell, C., Mihm, M.C., Hall, B.J., Chisholm, C., Jessup, C., Merola, M. (2014). Viral Infections. In: Dermatopathology. Springer, London. pp 239–251. https://doi.org/10.1007/978-1-4471-5448-8_17

8.12 Cockerell, C., Mihm, M.C., Hall, B.J., Chisholm, C., Jessup, C., Merola, M. (2014). Vascular Neoplasms and Malformations. In: Dermatopathology. Springer, London. pp 339–359. https://doi.org/10.1007/978-1-4471-5448-8_24

8.13 Cockerell, C., Mihm, M.C., Hall, B.J., Chisholm, C., Jessup, C., Merola, M. (2014). Fibrohistiocytic Neoplasms. In: Dermatopathology. Springer, London. pp 361–395. https://doi.org/10.1007/978-1-4471-5448-8_25

8.14 Cockerell, C., Mihm, M.C., Hall, B.J., Chisholm, C., Jessup, C., Merola, M. (2014). Metabolic and Depositional Disorders. In: Dermatopathology. Springer, London. pp 127–138. https://doi.org/10.1007/978-1-4471-5448-8_8

8.17 Phung, T.L., Wright, T.S., Pourciau, C.Y., Smoller, B.R. (2017). Papulosquamous Diseases. In: Pediatric Dermatopathology. Springer, Cham. pp 23–59. https://doi.org/10.1007/978-3-319-44824-4_2

8.20 Cockerell, C., Mihm, M.C., Hall, B.J., Chisholm, C., Jessup, C., Merola, M. (2014). Soft Tissue Neoplasms (Fat, Muscle). In: Dermatopathology. Springer, London. pp 397–412. https://doi.org/10.1007/978-1-4471-5448-8_26

8.23 Jain, S., Apichai, S.P. (2017). Pathology. In: Dermatology. Springer, Cham. pp 345–373. https://doi.org/10.1007/978-3-319-47395-6_8. (*Courtesy of* Dr. Euphemia Mu and Dr. Sheehan Meehan, NYU Dept. of Dermatology.)

8.24 Phung, T.L., Wright, T.S., Pourciau, C.Y., Smoller, B.R. (2017). Panniculitis. In: Pediatric Dermatopathology. Springer, Cham. pp 197–208. https://doi.org/10.1007/978-3-319-44824-4_9

8.25 Phung, T.L., Wright, T.S., Pourciau, C.Y., Smoller, B.R. (2017). Dermatoses with Minimal Epidermal Changes. In: Pediatric Dermatopathology. Springer, Cham. pp 121–139. https://doi.org/10.1007/978-3-319-44824-4_5

8.26 Phung, T.L., Wright, T.S., Pourciau, C.Y., Smoller, B.R. (2017). Fungal Diseases. In: Pediatric Dermatopathology. Springer, Cham. pp 279–297. https://doi.org/10.1007/978-3-319-44824-4_13

8.27 Phung, T.L., Wright, T.S., Pourciau, C.Y., Smoller, B.R. (2017). Fungal Diseases. In: Pediatric Dermatopathology. Springer, Cham. pp 279–297. https://doi.org/10.1007/978-3-319-44824-4_13

8.28 Jain, S., Apichai, S.P. (2017). Pathology. In: Dermatology. Springer, Cham. pp 345–373. https://doi.org/10.1007/978-3-319-47395-6_8. (*Courtesy of* Dr. Euphemia Mu and Dr. Sheehan Meehan, NYU Dept. of Dermatology.)

8.29 Phung, T.L., Wright, T.S., Pourciau, C.Y., Smoller, B.R. (2017). Fibrous Proliferations. In: Pediatric Dermatopathology. Springer, Cham. pp 529–553. https://doi.org/10.1007/978-3-319-44824-4_25

8.30 Phung, T.L., Wright, T.S., Pourciau, C.Y., Smoller, B.R. (2017). Deposition Disorders. In: Pediatric Dermatopathology. Springer, Cham. pp 317–345. https://doi.org/10.1007/978-3-319-44824-4_16

8.31 Phung, T.L., Wright, T.S., Pourciau, C.Y., Smoller, B.R. (2017). Adipocyte Proliferations. In: Pediatric Dermatopathology. Springer, Cham. pp 567–572. https://doi.org/10.1007/978-3-319-44824-4_27

8.32 Phung, T.L., Wright, T.S., Pourciau, C.Y., Smoller, B.R. (2017). Benign Hamartomatous Proliferations. In: Pediatric Dermatopathology. Springer, Cham. https://doi.org/10.1007/978-3-319-44824-4_29

8.34 Phung, T.L., Wright, T.S., Pourciau, C.Y., Smoller, B.R. (2017). Keratinous Cysts and Hamartomas. In: Pediatric Dermatopathology. Springer, Cham. https://doi.org/10.1007/978-3-319-44824-4_23

8.35 Cockerell, C., Mihm, M.C., Hall, B.J., Chisholm, C., Jessup, C., Merola, M. (2014). Adnexal Neoplasms. In: Dermatopathology. Springer, London. pp 425–467. https://doi.org/10.1007/978-1-4471-5448-8_28

1. **The dermoscopic image shows crypts and milia-like cysts. What are additional dermoscopic findings you may see with this diagnosis?**

2. **This dermoscopic image is most consistent with which of the following?**

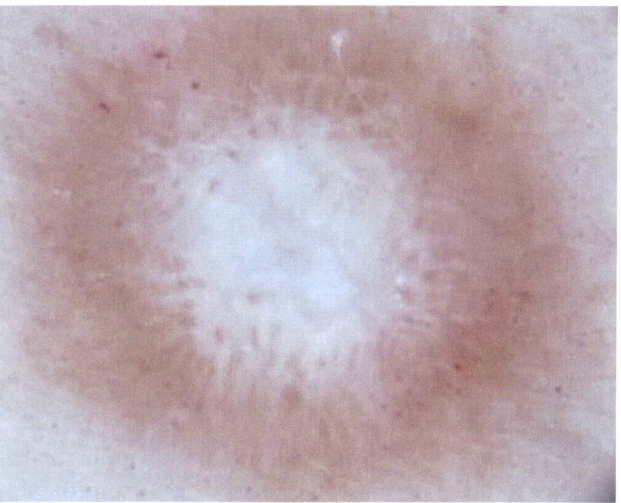

    (a) Seborrheic keratosis
    (b) Lentigo
    (c) Dermatofibroma
    (d) Acral nevus

    (a) Pseudopods
    (b) Blue-white veil
    (c) Spoke wheel-like structures
    (d) "Fat fingers" or gyri of a cerebriform surface

3. **This dermoscopic image shows characteristic dotted vessels arranged in a linear or serpiginous pattern. What is the diagnosis?**

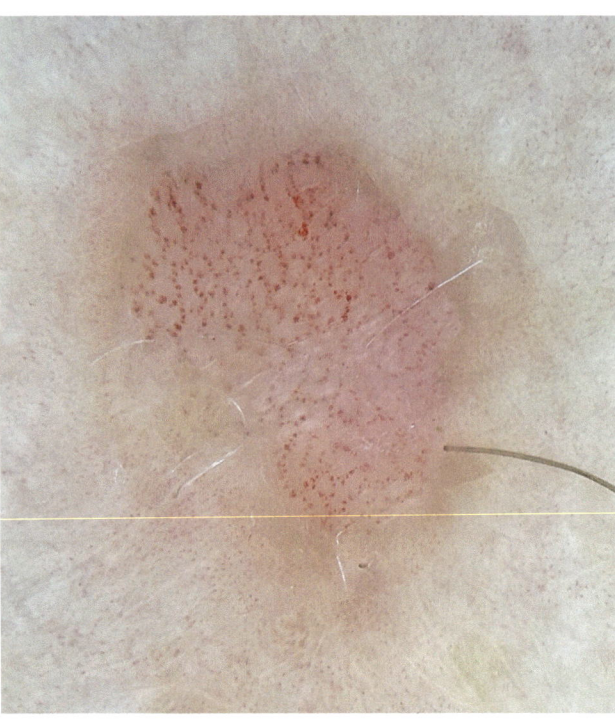

(a) Clear cell acanthoma
(b) Inverted follicular keratosis
(c) Syringoma
(d) Cylindroma

4. **A patient presents with yellow to pink papules on his face and the dermoscopic image is shown in the figure. What is the most likely diagnosis?**

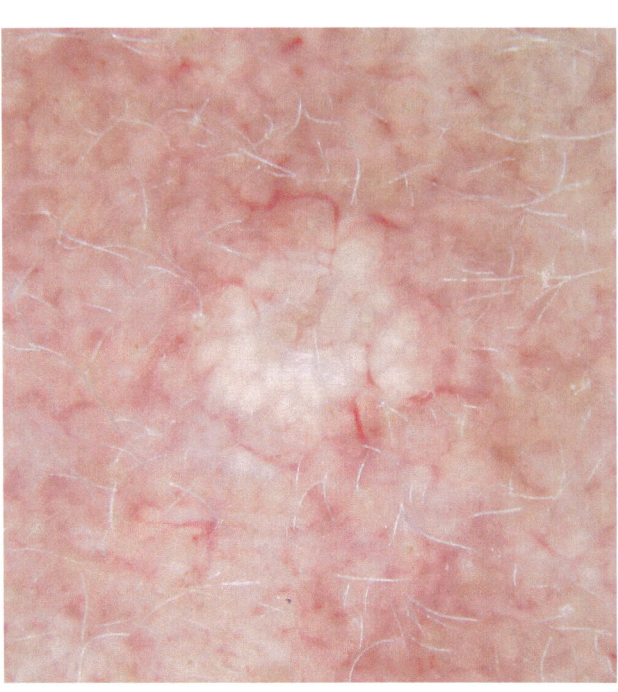

(a) Basal cell carcinoma
(b) Sebaceous hyperplasia
(c) Keratoacanthoma
(d) Dermal nevus

5. **This dermoscopic image was taken from a 22-year-old male with an erythematous scaly thin plaque on his elbow. The uniform distribution of red dots in the picture is representative of what feature histologically?**

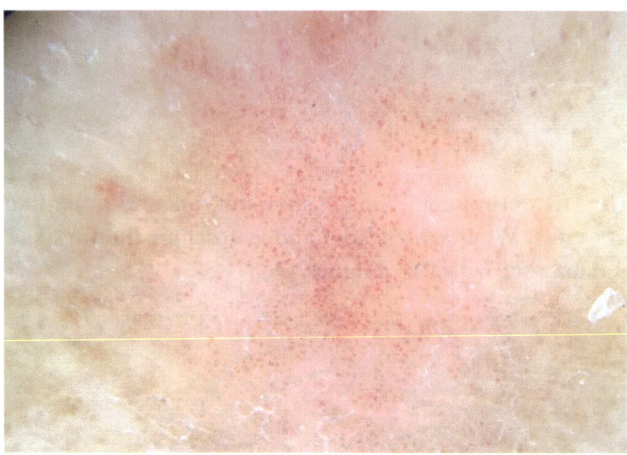

(a) Corresponds with the loops of vertically arranged vessels within the elongated dermal papillae in psoriasis
(b) Corresponds with the pink vessels in the normal dermal plexus within elongated dermal papillae in a fixed drug eruption
(c) Corresponds with horizontal dilated loops within the reticular dermis in psoriasis
(d) Corresponds with glomerular or coiled vessels in the elongated dermal papillae in lichen planus

6. **The dermoscopic findings of a "moth-eaten" edge and "fingerprint" pattern are seen typically in which of the following?**

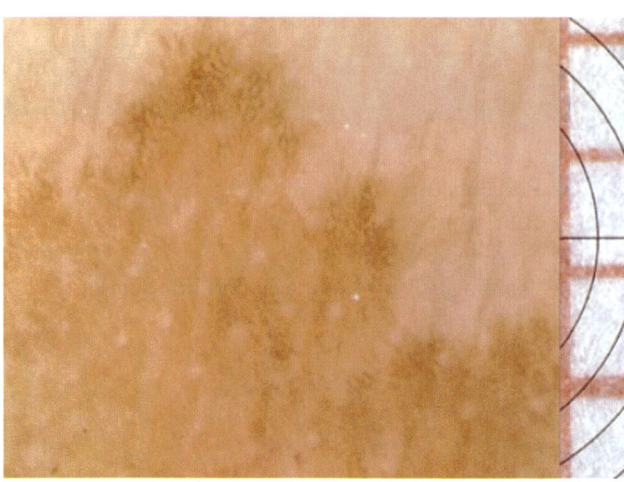

(a) Seborrheic keratosis
(b) Solar lentigo
(c) Dermatofibroma
(d) Nevus

7. **Polygonal vessels as seen in this dermoscopic image is most indicative of which of the following?**

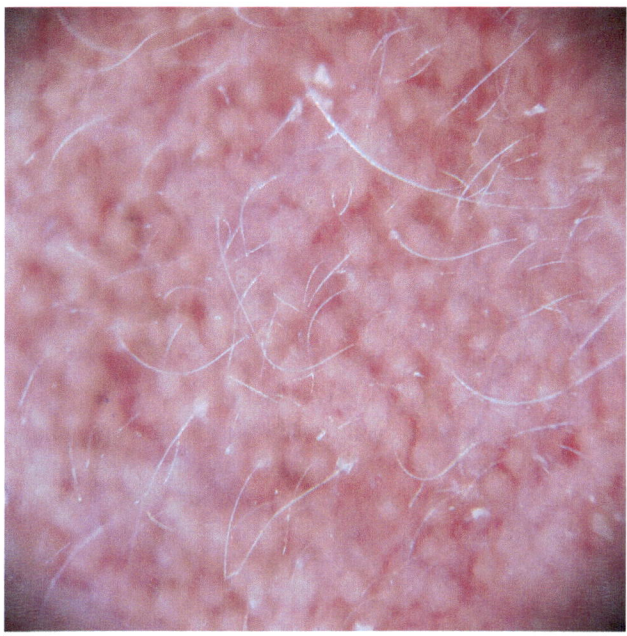

(a) Sarcoidosis
(b) Rosacea
(c) Contact dermatitis
(d) Psoriasis

8. **What is the most likely diagnosis of the dermoscopic image?**

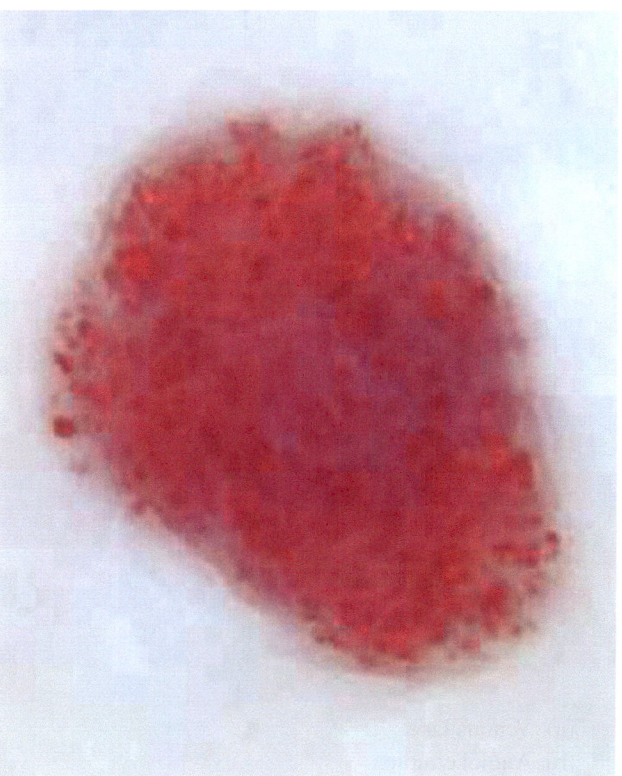

(a) Angioma
(b) Amelanotic melanoma
(c) Pyogenic granuloma
(d) Angiokeratoma

9. **The lesion in the figure is partial blanching (approximately 90%) with pressure. What is the most likely diagnosis?**

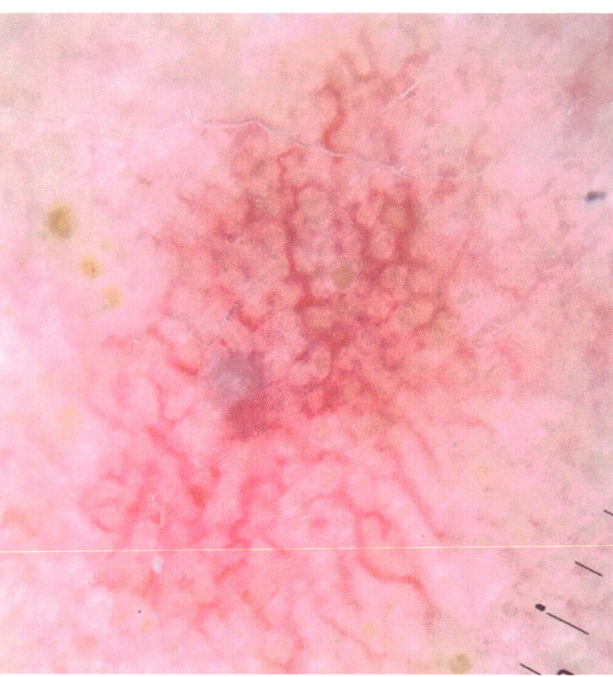

(a) Venous lake
(b) Angiokeratoma
(c) Spider angioma
(d) Amelanotic melanoma

10. **What are the dermoscopic signs that are consistent with the discoloration seen on the lateral toe in the figure?**

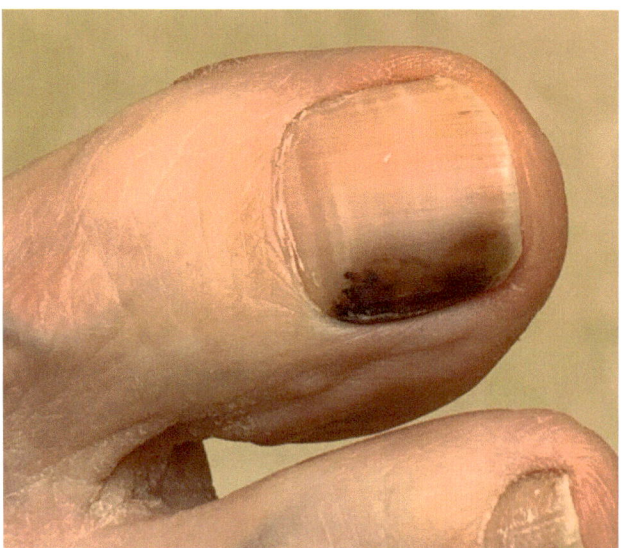

(a) Parallel furrow pattern
(b) Red-black homogenous pigmentation with satellite globules
(c) Pseudopods
(d) Pigmentation on the ridges of the surface skin markings

11. **What is the most likely diagnosis of this dermoscopic image?**

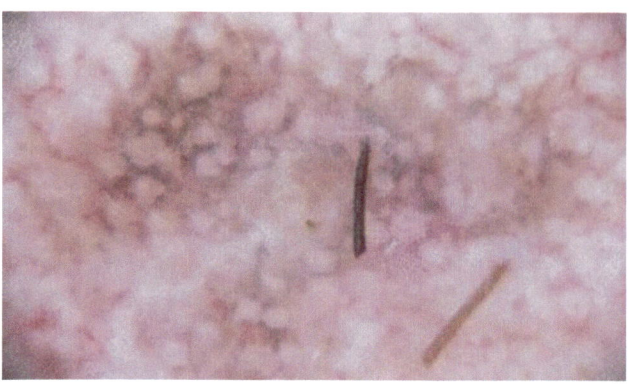

(a) Pigmented actinic keratosis
(b) Solar lentigo
(c) Ephelis
(d) Macular seborrheic keratosis

12. **What is the pattern shown in the dermoscopic image of this acral nevus? The area was inked with purple surgical marker and then wiped off with isopropyl alcohol.**

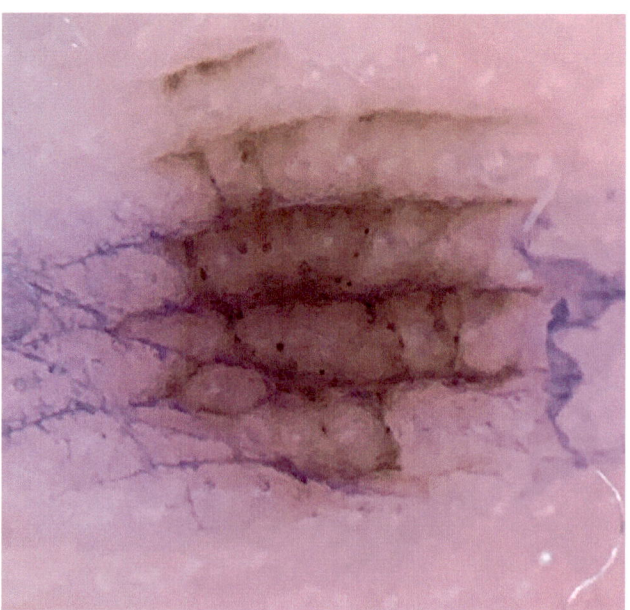

(a) Parallel ridge pattern
(b) Parallel furrow pattern
(c) Fibrillar pattern
(d) Lattice like pattern

13. **Common warts have all of the following features except:**
    (a) Homogenous black to red dots and globules over a white or light brown background
    (b) Central red dot or loop surrounded by whitish halo with a 'frogspawn' appearance
    (c) Abrupt interruption of the natural dermatoglyphics
    (d) A central area with white and/or yellow amorphous structures and a peripheral crown of linear or branched vessels

14. **The virus that typically causes the changes shown in the figure is:**

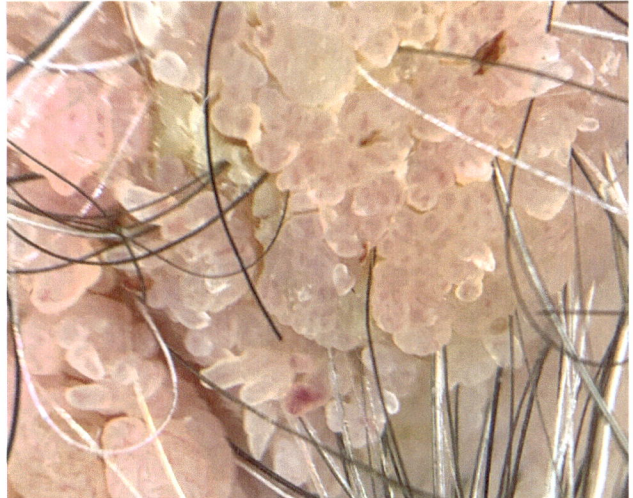

    (a) Human papilloma virus
    (b) Pox virus
    (c) Herpes simplex virus
    (d) Varicella zoster virus

15. **The virus that causes the lesions shown in the figure is:**

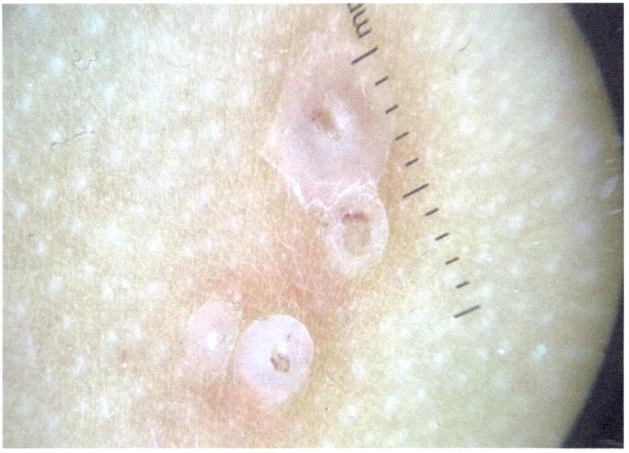

    (a) Molluscum contagiosum virus (pox virus)
    (b) Human papilloma virus
    (c) Herpes simplex virus
    (d) Varicella zoster virus

16. **Which of the following is not true regarding the dermoscopic findings you would see in scabies?**

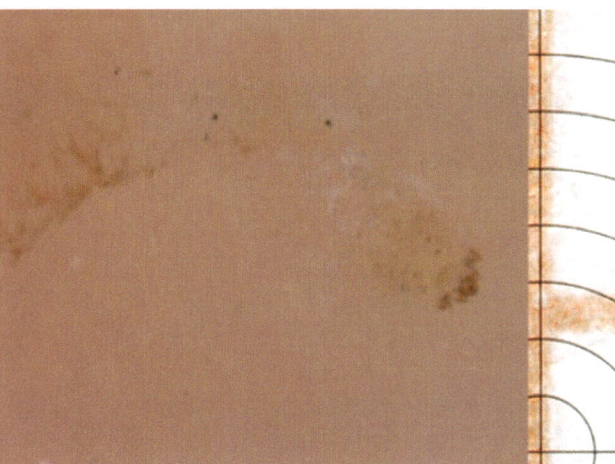

    (a) The burrow typically shows a small dark brown triangular structure (delta wing jet or mini triangle sign) located at the end of a whitish structureless lines ("jet contrail")
    (b) The brown triangle represents the mite but correlates specifically with the pigmented anterior portion of the mite and the rest of the body of the mite shows up as relatively translucent
    (c) The whitish structureless lines (jet "contrail") contain the eggs and feces
    (d) The mite is not visible on dermoscopy and the brown triangle indicates a cluster of feces

17. **This dermoscopic image is from the nail fold and the capillaries are focally dilated and tortuous. Which of the following is the least likely condition you might see this in?**

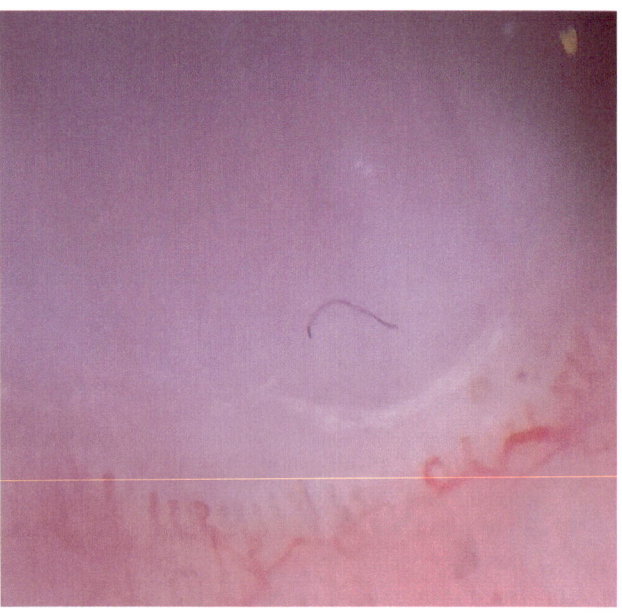

   (a) Lupus erythematosus
   (b) Dermatomyositis
   (c) Scleroderma
   (d) Lichen planus

18. **Significant follicular plugging showing a "carpet tack" sign, telangiectasia and pigment drop is most commonly seen with which of the following?**

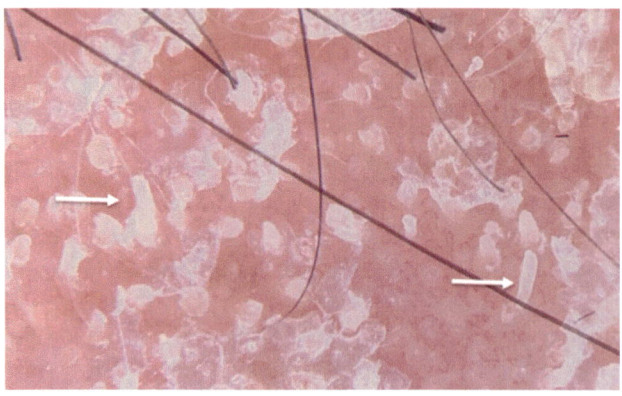

   (a) Discoid lupus erythematosus
   (b) Lichen planus
   (c) Pigmented actinic keratosis
   (d) Fixed drug eruption

19. **This 55-year-old woman presents with a 2-year history of an erythematous plaque on her cheek. The dermoscopic image shows a localized structureless area with a yellowish-orange or apply-jelly color. What is the most likely diagnosis?**

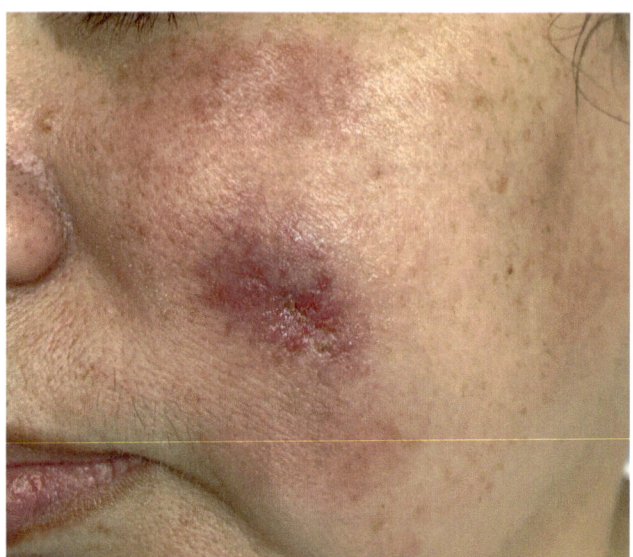

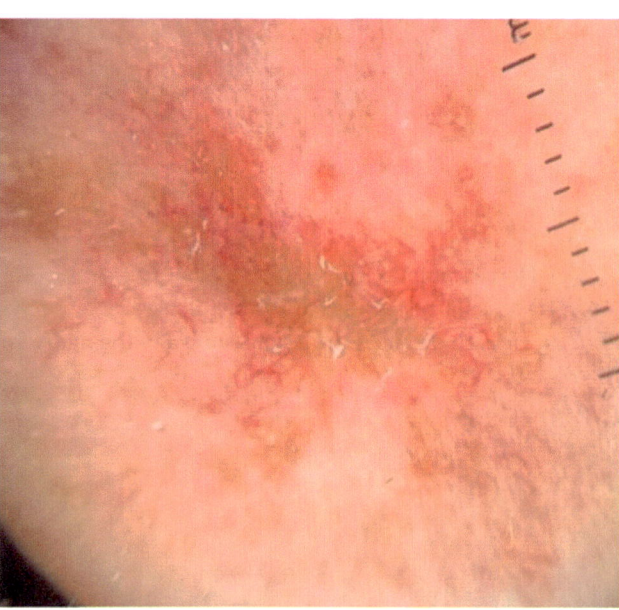

   (a) Sarcoidosis
   (b) Discoid lupus erythematosus
   (c) Sweet syndrome
   (d) Impetigo

20. **Arborizing vessels are most consistently seen with:**

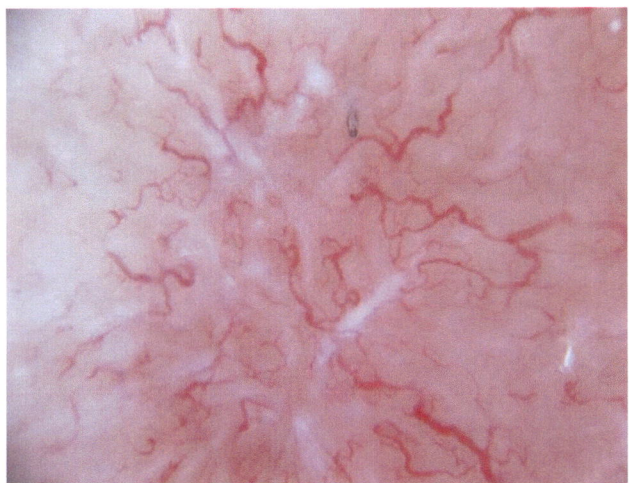

    (a) Basal cell carcinoma
    (b) Squamous cell carcinoma
    (c) Bowen's disease
    (d) Amelanotic melanoma

21. **The most likely diagnosis of this dermoscopic image is:**

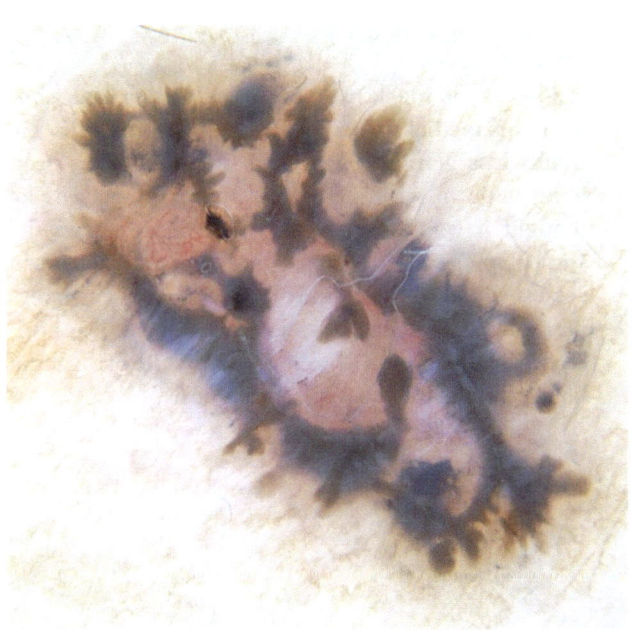

    (a) Melanoma
    (b) Basal cell carcinoma
    (c) Pigmented Bowen's disease
    (d) Dysplastic nevus

22. **What is the most important feature to help distinguish this pigmented basal cell from a melanoma?**

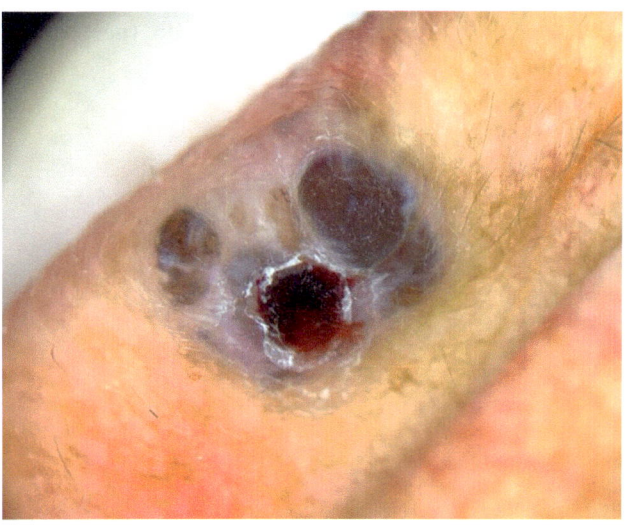

    (a) Lack of a pigment network
    (b) Lack of orthogonal white lines
    (c) Lack of dilated tortuous vessels
    (d) Lack of blue-white veil

23. **The dermoscopic finding pictured in the figure will most likely correlate with which of the following histopathologic findings?**

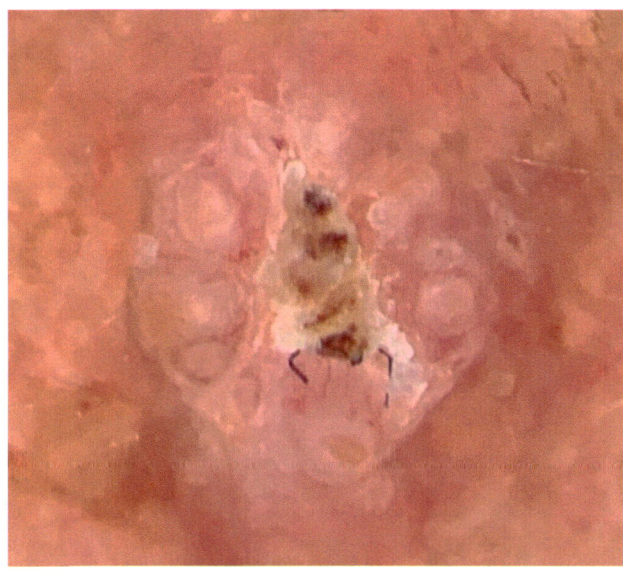

    (a) Keratin pearls in a well-differentiated squamous cell carcinoma
    (b) Dilated tortuous vessels in a basal cell carcinoma
    (c) Crown vessels in sebaceous hyperplasia
    (d) Thrombosed central vessel in verruca vulgaris

24. **A patient presents with a new lesion for the past 5 months on the chest and the dermoscopic image is shown in the figure. Which of the following is a dermoscopic feature not associated with the type of tumor?**

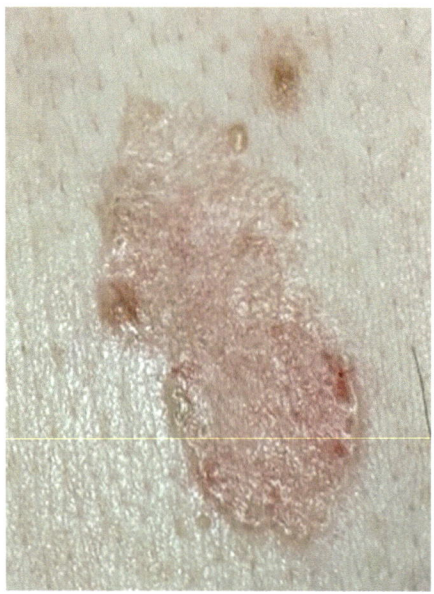

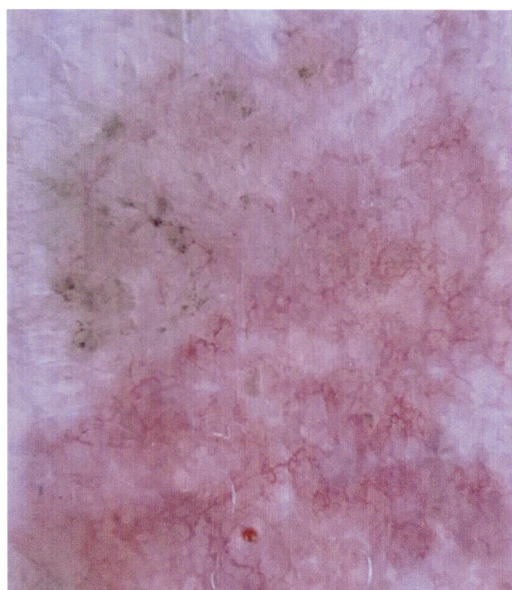

(a) Blue-gray ovoid nests and dots/globules
(b) Maple leaf-like areas and spoke wheel-like structures
(c) Arborizing vessels and superficial fine telangiectasias
(d) Ulceration and multiple small erosions
(e) Glomerular (coiled) vessels and dotted vessels

25. **Which of the following is not a feature seen in the melanoma pictured in the figure?**

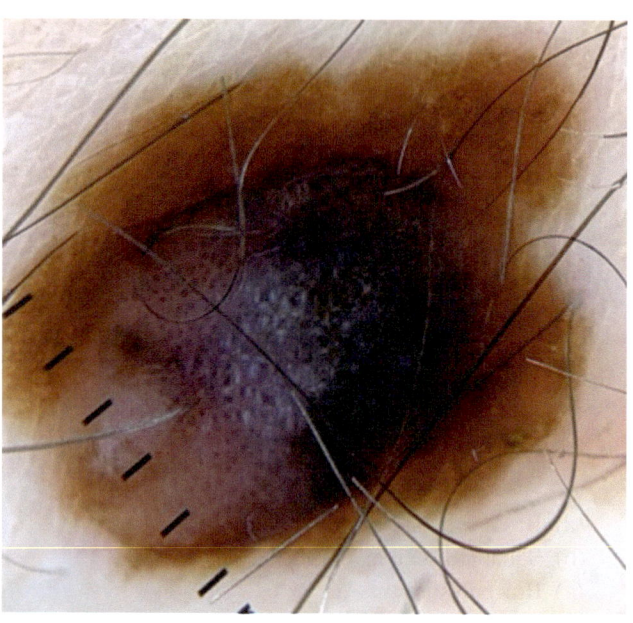

(a) Negative pigment network
(b) Multitude of colors
(c) Orthogonal white lines
(d) Pseudopods

26. **A 34-year-old black male presented with a pink papule to his medial malleolus for the past 3 months. He thinks it is getting bigger and the patient has been filing it down with a pumice stone regularly as he thought it was just a callus. This figure shows the clinical image. On dermoscopic exam, polymorphous vessels with a combination of dotted and linear irregular and a few helical vessels are seen. There are different shades of pink as well as a few white orthogonal lines. What is the most likely diagnosis?**

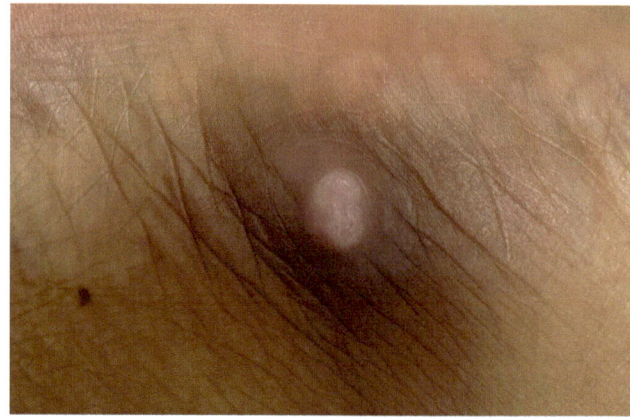

(a) Pyogenic granuloma
(b) Exuberant granulation tissue from constant trauma
(c) Hypertrophic scar
(d) Amelanotic melanoma

27. **Which of the following dermoscopic finding is least likely to be seen in the type of lesion pictured in the figure?**

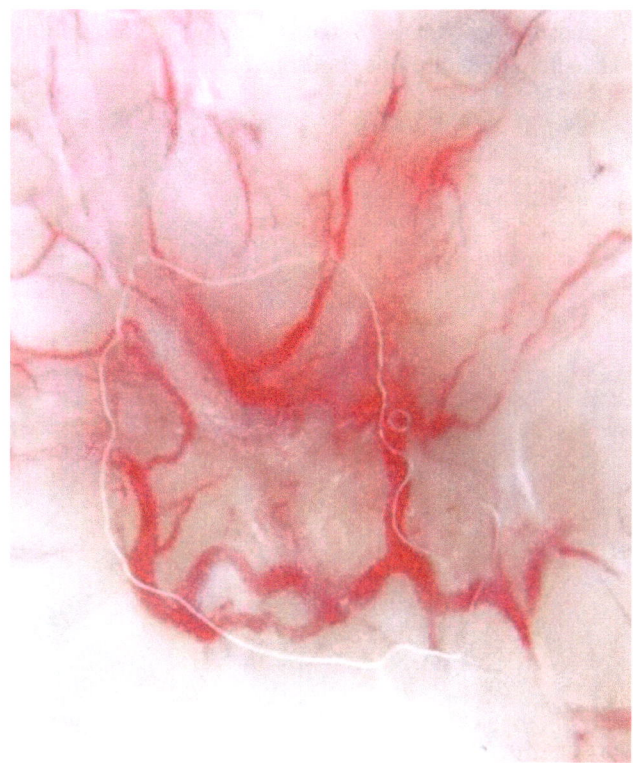

(a) Spoke wheel-like structures
(b) Maple leaf-like areas
(c) Ulceration
(d) Orthogonal white lines
(e) Negative pigment network

28. **The dermoscopic feature of regular glomerular vessels with focal ulceration is most consistent with which of the following?**

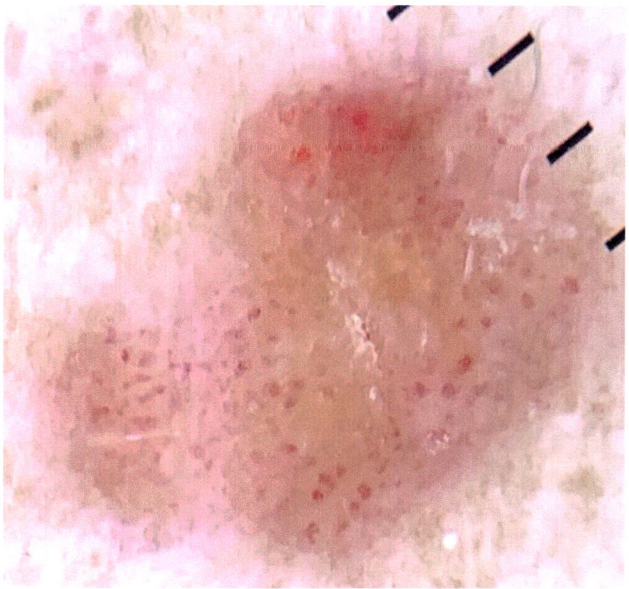

(a) Bowen's disease
(b) Squamous cell carcinoma
(c) Inflamed seborrheic keratosis
(d) Amelanotic melanoma

29. **The most likely diagnosis for the dermoscopic image in this 75-year-old male with a brown area on the tip of his nose for the past 2 years is which of the following?**

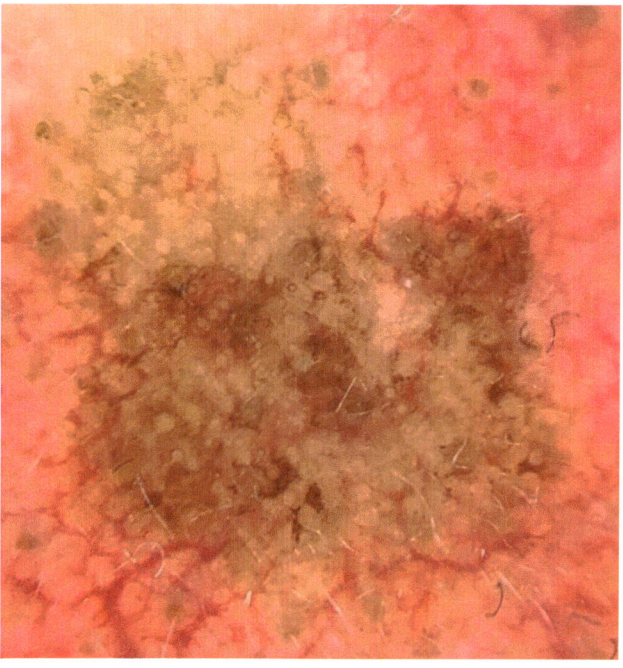

(a) Lentigo
(b) Seborrheic keratosis
(c) Melanoma in situ
(d) Ephelis

30. **A 45-year-old female complains of hair loss for the past 2 months that she says involves all of her scalp. She denies any irritation, itching or pain to the affected areas. The patient denies any new medications before the onset of hair loss, but she does state that she had a positive COVID-19 infection about 4 months ago. This figure shows the dermoscopic image. What is most likely the cause?**

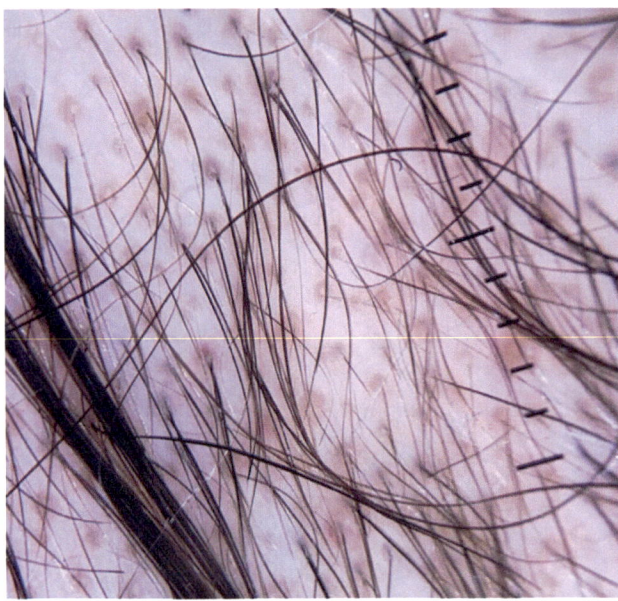

   (a) Telogen effluvium
   (b) Androgenetic alopecia
   (c) Trichotillomania
   (d) Lichen planopilaris

31. **A 48-year-old female comes to your office for hair loss that is gradually been worsening for the past 3 years with a widening part line. She denies any itching or soreness to the scalp. This figure shows the dermoscopic image. What is the most helpful finding to help diagnose this condition?**

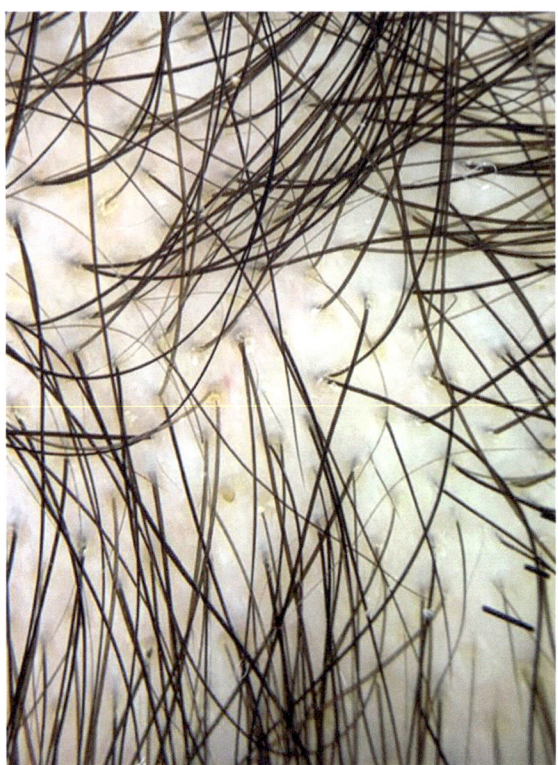

   (a) The variation in hair shaft diameter is less than 10% on dermoscopic exam
   (b) There is mild perifollicular scale
   (c) The variation in hair shaft diameter is greater than 20% on dermoscopic exam
   (d) There is perifollicular subtle hyperpigmentation

32. **A 23-year-old female with a history of obsessive-compulsive disorder comes with hair loss. The clinical photo is to the left and the dermoscopic image is to the right. She adamantly denies any pulling of her hair. What is the most likely diagnosis?**

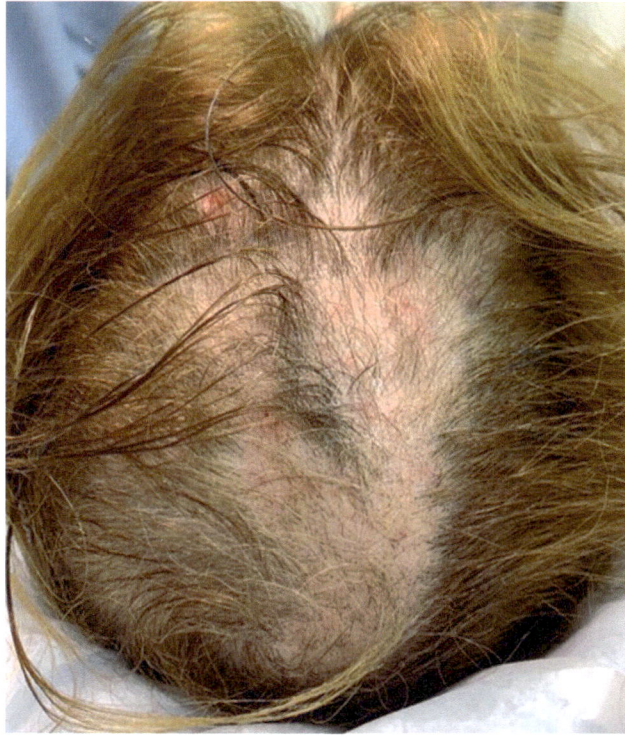

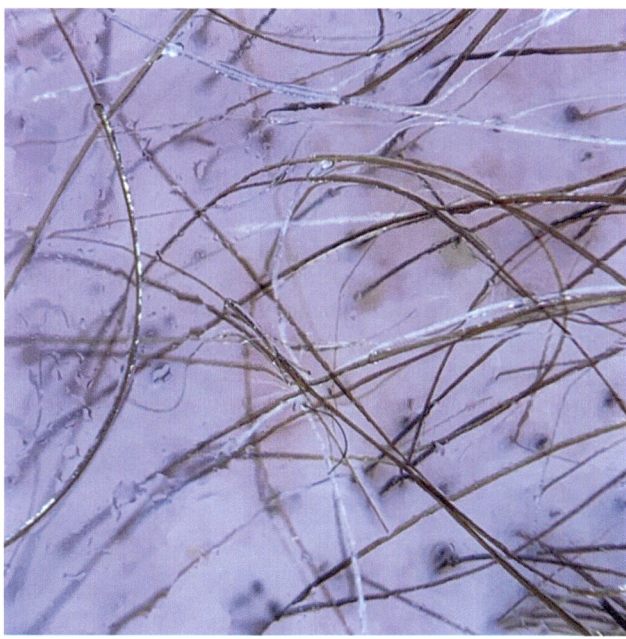

(a) Trichotillomania
(b) Alopecia areata
(c) Androgenetic alopecia
(d) Pressure-induced alopecia

33. **A 45-year-old female has noticed small bumps on her forehead for the past 1 year. On further questioning, she admits to her forehead appearing bigger over the past year but is not sure if she has noticed hair loss. On dermoscopic exam of the frontal hairline, you notice peripilar scale and surrounding subtle erythema. What is the most likely diagnosis?**

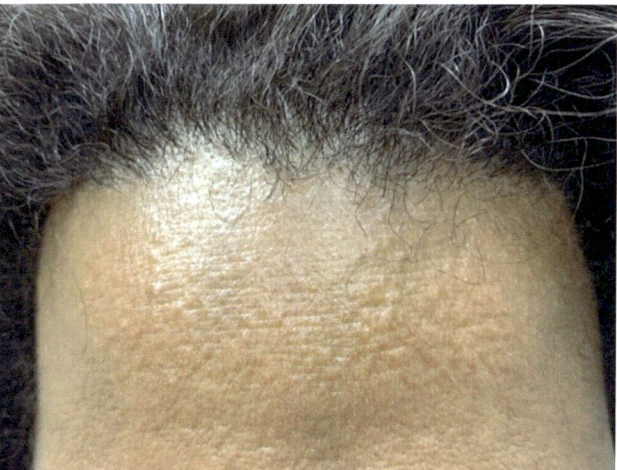

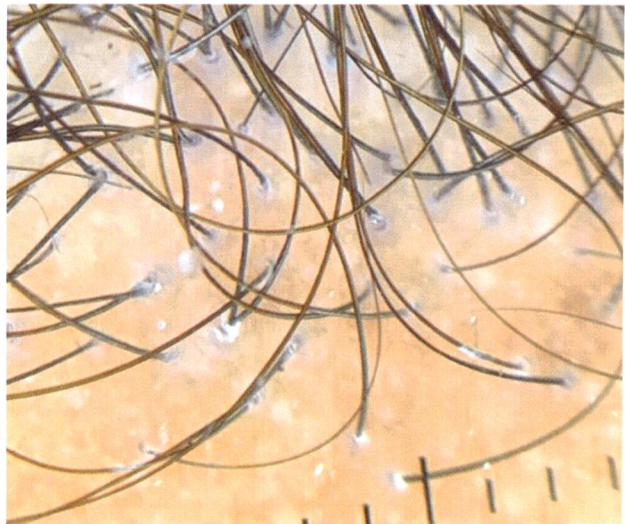

(a) Central centrifugal cicatricial alopecia (CCCA)
(b) Alopecia areata
(c) Traction alopecia
(d) Frontal fibrosing alopecia (FFA)

34. **A 25-year-old female comes in for a flare of alopecia areata. The original clinical photo is shown to the left. It was treated with an intralesional triamcinolone at her last visit and she comes back today. Her follow up dermoscopic image is shown to the right. What are the dermoscopic features that show alopecia areata is still active and needs to be treated again? There are two answer choices that are correct.**

   (a) Black dots
   (b) Exclamation mark (tapered) hairs
   (c) Yellow dots
   (d) Peripilar sign

35. **The dermoscopic image from a hair loss patient shows perifollicular scaling in a background of erythema with loss of follicular ostia. This is most likely diagnosis is which of the following?**

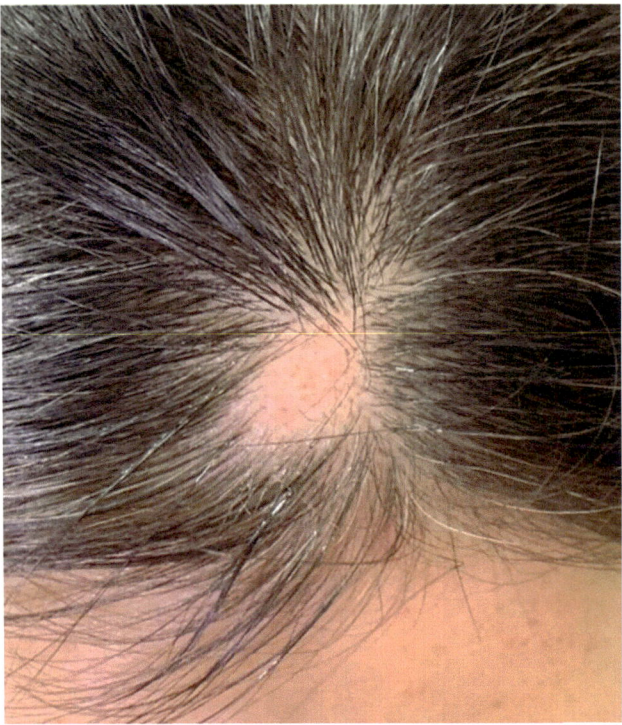

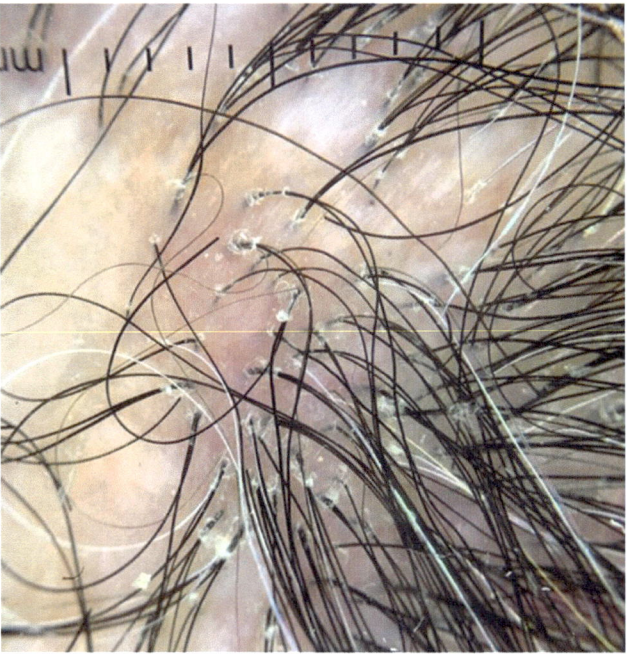

   (a) Lichen planopilaris (LPP)
   (b) Androgenetic alopecia
   (c) Telogen effluvium
   (d) Frontal fibrosing alopecia
   (e) Central centrifugal cicatricial alopecia (CCCA)

Answer Key

For further information regarding the below answers, please see Chapter 9 of the corresponding *Dermatology: Illustrated Study Guide and Comprehensive Board Review, 3rd Edition* (2024).

   1. **d**
   2. **c**
   3. **a**
   4. **b**
   5. **a**
   6. **b**
   7. **b**
   8. **a**
   9. **c**
   10. **b**
   11. **a**

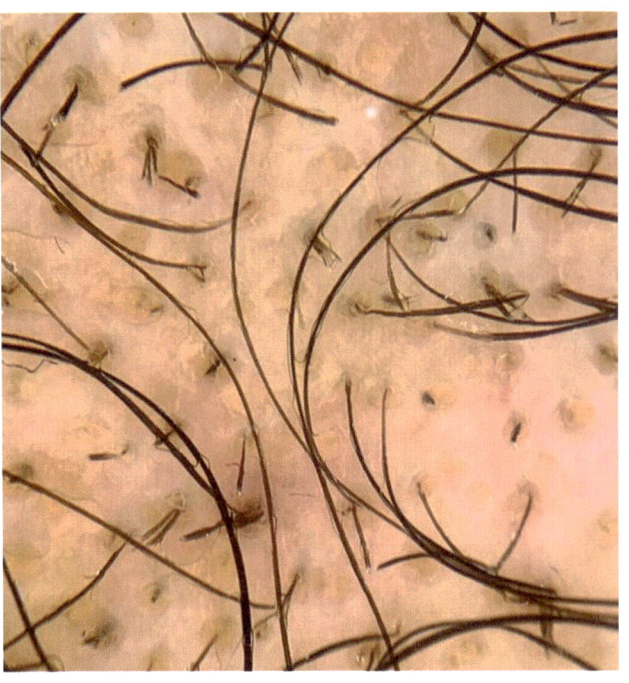

12. **b**

13. **d**

14. **a**

15. **a**

16. **d**

17. **d**

18. **a**

19. **a**

20. **a**

21. **b**

22. **a**

23. **a**

24. **e**

25. **d**

26. **d**

27. **e**

28. **a**

29. **c**

30. **a**

31. **c**

32. **a**

33. **d**

34. **a and b**

35. **a**

Image Sources

9.1 Jain, S. (2017). Dermoscopy and Electron Microscopy. In: Dermatology. Springer, Cham. pp 375–388. https://doi.org/10.1007/978-3-319-47395-6_9

9.3 *Courtesy of* Curtis Asbury, MD.

9.6 Schulz H, Argenyi A, Gambichler T, Altmeyer P, Paech V. S. In: Compendium of Surface Microscopic and Dermoscopic Features. Berlin, Heidelberg: Springer; 2008. https://doi.org/10.1007/978-3-540-78973-4_18

9.11 Jain, S. (2017). Dermoscopy and Electron Microscopy. In: Dermatology. Springer, Cham. pp 375–388 https://doi.org/10.1007/978-3-319-47395-6_9

9.16 (2008). S. In: Compendium of Surface Microscopic and Dermoscopic Features. Springer, Berlin, Heidelberg. https://doi.org/10.1007/978-3-540-78973-4_18

9.27 Jain, S. (2017). Dermoscopy and Electron Microscopy. In: Dermatology. Springer, Cham. pp 375–388 https://doi.org/10.1007/978-3-319-47395-6_9

Index

© The Editor(s) (if applicable) and The Author(s), under exclusive license to Springer Nature Switzerland AG 2024
S. Jain, *Dermatology High-Yield Self-Assessment*, https://doi.org/10.1007/978-3-031-73263-8

GPSR Compliance

*The European Union's (EU) General Product Safety Regulation (GPSR)
is a set of rules that requires consumer products to be safe and our
obligations to ensure this.*

*If you have any concerns about our products, you can contact us on
ProductSafety@springernature.com*

In case Publisher is established outside the EU, the EU authorized
representative is:

Springer Nature Customer Service Center GmbH
Europaplatz 3
69115 Heidelberg, Germany

Batch number: 09640318

Printed by Printforce, the Netherlands